Energy Medicine Unlocked

A Comprehensive Guide to Healing

Mei Lin Zhang

Xspurts.com

A New Zealand Designed Product

Other Versions Available

Why limit yourself to just one format?

This book is now available in physical, digital, and audiobook options.

Choose the way you love to read and dive into the story today. You won't regret it!

Digital ISBN: 9781776849710
Physical ISBN: 9781776849048
Audio ISBN:

To obtain a different format of this book at a discounted price, please get in touch with us at:

http://isbn.xspurts.com/

Contents

Have Questions / Comments?

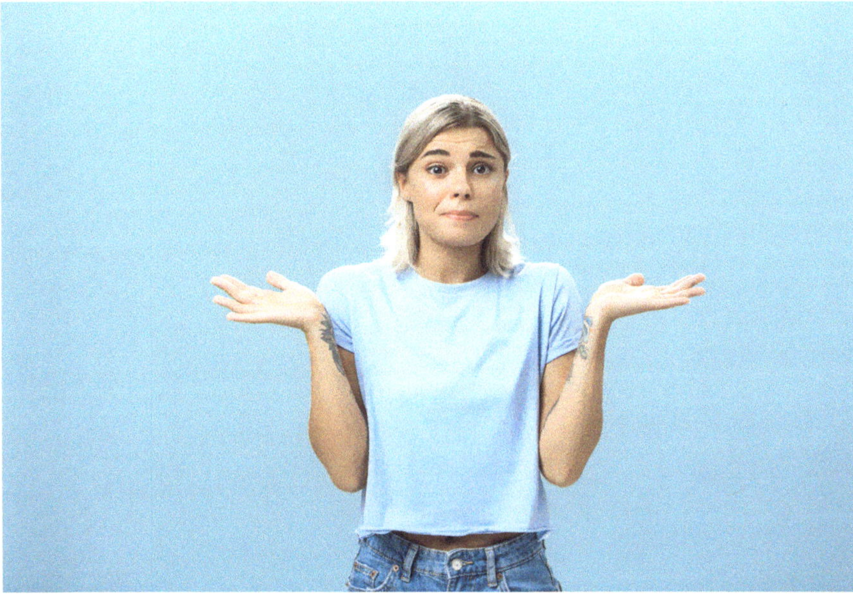

This book was designed to cover as much information as possible, but I know I have probably missed something, or some new amazing discovery has just come out.

If you notice something missing or have a question that I failed to answer, please get in touch and let me know. If I can, I will email you an answer and also update the book so others can also benefit from it.

Thanks For Being Awesome :)

Submit Your Questions / Comments At:

https://questions.xspurts.com

Get Free Stuff

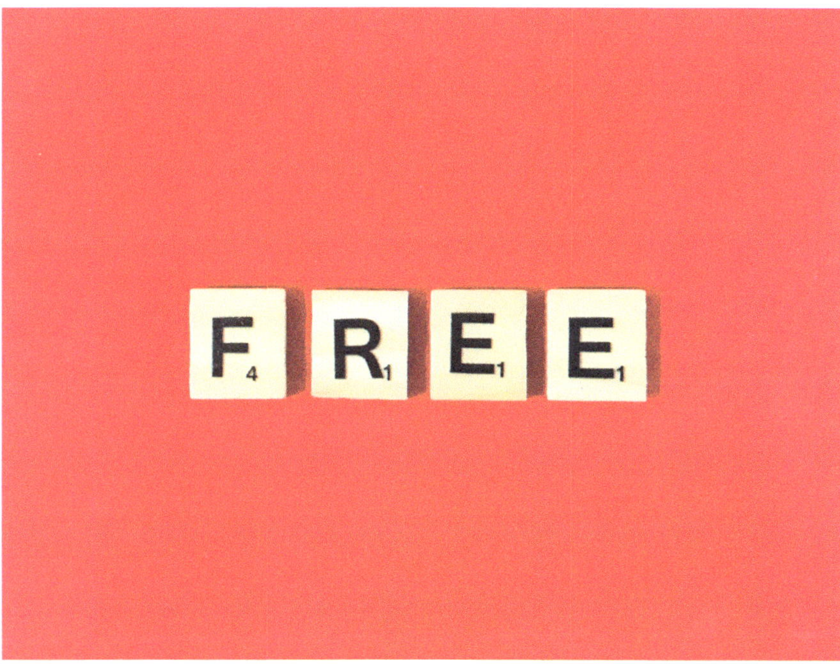

We love writing and have produced a huge number of books.

For being one of our amazing readers, we would love to offer you more books we have created, 100% free.

To claim this limited time special offer, simply go to the site below and enter your name and email address.

You will then receive loads (as we love our readers so much :) of our great books, content and audio direct to your email account, 100% free!

Get Loads of FREE Stuff at:

https://free.xspurts.com

Chapter One

Understanding Energy Medicine

In the quest for health and well-being, humans have explored various forms of medicine throughout history. From ancient healing practices to modern advancements, the field of medicine has evolved significantly. One intriguing branch of alternative medicine that has gained attention in recent years is energy medicine. This holistic approach recognizes the role of energy in promoting health and treating ailments. Below we will delve into the fascinating world of energy medicine, exploring its principles, techniques, and potential benefits.

Energy medicine is based on the belief that the human body is composed of a complex network of energy systems that interact and influence our well-being. These energy systems include meridians, chakras, and auras, among others. Practitioners of energy medicine focus on balancing and optimizing the flow of energy within these systems to promote physical, emotional, and spiritual health.

One widely recognized aspect of energy medicine is acupuncture, which originated in ancient China thousands of years ago. Acupuncture involves the insertion of thin needles into specific points along the body's meridians to correct imbalances and restore the flow of energy. Scientific studies have shown that acupuncture can stimulate the release of endorphins, promote circulation, and reduce pain. It has been successfully used to treat various conditions such as chronic pain, migraines, and even addiction.

Another well-known energy healing practice is Reiki. Developed in Japan in the late 19th century, Reiki involves the transfer of healing energy through the practitioner's hands to the recipient. The practitioner acts as a channel, directing the universal life force energy to areas of the body that need healing. Reiki is known for inducing deep relaxation, reducing stress, and supporting the body's natural healing processes. While the scientific evidence for Reiki is still limited, many individuals report significant improvements in their overall well-being after receiving Reiki treatments.

Crystals are also utilized in energy medicine for their unique vibrational properties. Each crystal is believed to emit a specific energy frequency that can interact with the body's energy field. Different crystals are associated with various healing properties, such as rose quartz for promoting love and self-acceptance or amethyst for calming the mind and enhancing spiritual connection. Crystal therapy involves placing crystals on or around the body to restore balance and harmony.

Sound healing is another modality used in energy medicine. The use of sound vibrations to promote healing dates back thousands of years and can be found in many cultural and spiritual traditions. Sound healing can involve chanting, singing bowls, or the use of specific frequencies to entrain the body's energy systems. Studies have shown that sound therapy can reduce stress, lower blood pressure, and improve sleep quality. It is particularly effective in inducing deep relaxation and facilitating meditation.

Energy medicine also encompasses practices such as qigong, tai chi, and yoga, which combine movement, breath control, and focused intention to balance and harmonize the body's energy systems. These ancient practices have been shown to improve flexibility, strength, and overall well-being. They help to cultivate mindfulness and create a deeper connection between the mind, body, and spirit.

While energy medicine is often considered complementary to conventional medical treatments, it is essential to approach it with an open mind and seek qualified practitioners. As with any form of medicine, it is crucial to ensure the safety and expertise of those providing energy healing. It is also important to note that energy medicine should not replace traditional medical care but rather be used in conjunction with it.

The history and evolution of energy medicine

Throughout human history, the quest for health and healing has led to the development of diverse medical systems. Among these, energy medicine stands out as a unique approach that recognizes the vital role of energy in maintaining well-being. The roots of energy medicine can be traced back thousands of years, with its evolution reflecting the profound understanding of energy and its impact on the human body. Below we will explore the fascinating history and evolution of energy medicine, shedding light on its origins, key figures, and advancements.

Ancient civilizations, such as the Egyptians, Greeks, and Chinese, were among the early pioneers of energy medicine. These cultures recognized the existence of an energetic life force flowing through the body, referred to as qi, prana, or vital energy. They developed various practices to influence this energy and maintain its balance for optimal health.

In China, the foundation for energy medicine was laid with the development of acupuncture. Dating back over 2,500 years, acupuncture is based on the concept of meridians, channels through which vital energy flows. By inserting thin needles into specific points along these meridians, practitioners aimed to restore the harmonious flow of energy and promote healing. Acupuncture remains a prominent modality in energy medicine, gaining recognition and popularity worldwide.

1. Similarly, Ayurveda, the traditional medicine of India, incorporates the concept of energy in its healing practices. According to Ayurvedic philosophy, the body is composed of three doshas: Vata, Pitta, and Kapha. These doshas represent different combinations of energy and influence an individual's physical and mental constitution. Ayurvedic treatments, including herbal remedies, dietary adjustments, and lifestyle practices, aim to balance the doshas and restore optimal energy flow.

In the early 20th century, a pivotal figure emerged in the field of energy medicine—Dr. Wilhelm Reich. Reich, an Austrian psychiatrist, proposed the existence of a universal life force energy he called "orgone." He developed various devices, such as the orgone accumulator, to harness and direct this energy for healing purposes. Although his work faced controversy and skepticism, Reich's contributions laid the groundwork for future explorations in energy medicine.

Another significant milestone in the history of energy medicine came with the discovery and understanding of the human biofield. The biofield refers to the electromagnetic and subtle energy field surrounding and interpenetrating the human body. In the 20th century, researchers such as Harold Burr and Valerie Hunt conducted studies that shed light on the existence and influence of the biofield on health and well-being. Their work paved the way for a deeper understanding of energy medicine and its applications.

During the latter half of the 20th century, various energy healing modalities gained recognition and popularity. One notable practice is Reiki, developed in Japan by Mikao Usui in the late 19th century. Reiki involves the transfer of healing energy through the hands of a practitioner to the recipient. It focuses on balancing the body's energy centers, known as chakras, and promoting relaxation and well-being. Reiki has since been widely practiced and has gained acceptance in many healthcare settings.

Crystal therapy is another ancient practice that gained renewed interest in modern energy medicine. Crystals are believed to possess specific vibrational properties that can interact with the body's energy field. Different crystals are associated with various healing properties, and practitioners use them in various ways, such as placing them on the body or incorporating them into jewelry. Crystal therapy aims to restore energetic balance and promote healing and well-being.

Sound healing, also known as vibrational therapy, has roots in ancient civilizations and spiritual traditions worldwide. The use of sound, whether through vocal toning, chanting, or the use of specific instruments such as singing bowls or tuning forks, has

Basic concepts and principles

Energy medicine is a holistic approach to healing that recognizes the vital role of energy in the maintenance of health and well-being. It operates on the principle that the human body is not just a physical entity but also an intricate network of energy systems that influence our overall state of being. Understanding the basic concepts and principles of energy medicine is key to unlocking its potential for promoting health and facilitating healing. Below we will explore these fundamental concepts, shedding light on how energy flows within the body, the role of energy centers, and the principles that govern energy healing.

Central to energy medicine is the concept of energy flow. According to this principle, the human body is permeated by a complex network of energy channels through which life force energy, known as qi, prana, or vital energy, flows. These channels are often referred to as meridians, nadis, or energy pathways. The uninterrupted flow of energy is essential for maintaining physical, emotional, and spiritual well-being. Any disruption or blockage in these energy pathways can lead to imbalances and eventually manifest as illness or disease.

The energy centers, or chakras, are another key concept in energy medicine. Chakras are spinning wheels or vortexes of energy located at specific points along the body's midline. Each chakra is associated with different aspects of our being, such as physical vitality, emotional well-being, creativity, intuition, and spiritual connection. Energy practitioners focus on balancing and harmonizing the chakras to ensure a smooth flow of energy throughout the body. This is achieved through various techniques such as meditation, visualization, and hands-on healing.

One principle that underlies energy medicine is the interconnectedness of mind, body, and spirit. It recognizes that physical ailments are often intertwined with emotional and spiritual imbalances. Therefore, addressing the underlying energetic aspects of an issue can have a profound impact on overall well-being. Energy medicine seeks to promote a holistic understanding of health, where the interplay between the physical, emotional, and spiritual realms is acknowledged and addressed.

Intention and focused awareness play a crucial role in energy healing. The intention of the healer or practitioner, combined with the recipient's receptivity and intention to heal, sets the stage for energy work. By directing focused awareness and intention, practitioners can influence the flow of energy and facilitate the body's natural healing processes. This principle highlights the significance of the mind-body connection in energy medicine and emphasizes the importance of cultivating a positive and healing mindset.

Another key principle in energy medicine is the concept of resonance and entrainment. Resonance refers to the phenomenon where two energy systems with similar frequencies vibrate in harmony and amplify each other's energy. Entrainment, on the other hand, occurs when two energy systems come into close proximity, and the weaker system adjusts its frequency to match that of the stronger system. These principles explain how energy healing techniques, such as sound healing or hands-on healing, can positively influence the recipient's energy field and promote balance and well-being.

Energy medicine also acknowledges the existence of subtle energy fields surrounding the physical body. These fields, often referred to as the biofield or aura, are composed of electromagnetic energy and subtle vibrations. They interact with the physical body and serve as a blueprint or template for its functioning. The biofield provides valuable information about a person's energetic state and can be assessed and addressed in energy healing sessions.

It is important to note that energy medicine is complementary to conventional medical care and does not replace it. It is not meant to diagnose or treat specific medical conditions but rather to support the body's natural healing abilities and promote overall well-being. Energy medicine practitioners work in conjunction with healthcare professionals to provide holistic care to individuals.

The role of energy medicine in modern healthcare

In recent years, there has been a growing interest in alternative approaches to healthcare that focus on holistic well-being. One such approach is energy medicine, which recognizes the vital role of energy in maintaining health and promoting healing. While energy medicine was once considered on the fringes of healthcare, it is now gaining recognition and acceptance within modern medical settings. Below we will explore the role of energy medicine in modern healthcare, highlighting its benefits, applications, and integration with conventional medicine.

Energy medicine offers a unique perspective on health and healing by recognizing that the human body is not just a physical entity but also an intricate network of energy systems. It acknowledges that imbalances or blockages in these energy systems can contribute to physical, emotional, and spiritual ailments. By addressing the underlying energetic aspects of a condition, energy medicine aims to restore balance and promote well-being.

One significant area where energy medicine is making strides in modern healthcare is pain management. Chronic pain affects millions of people worldwide and often presents complex challenges in conventional medical treatments. Energy medicine techniques such as acupuncture, which targets the body's energy meridians, have shown promising results in alleviating pain and reducing reliance on pain medications. Studies have shown that acupuncture can stimulate the release of endorphins, natural pain-relieving chemicals in the body, and modulate the perception of pain.

Furthermore, energy medicine modalities like Reiki and therapeutic touch have gained recognition for their ability to induce deep relaxation and reduce stress, both of which have a significant impact on overall health. Stress is a contributing factor to many chronic conditions, including cardiovascular disease, immune dysfunction, and mental health disorders. By promoting relaxation and balancing the body's energy, energy medicine techniques can support the body's natural healing responses and help individuals manage stress-related symptoms.

Another area where energy medicine is finding its place in modern healthcare is in supporting mental health and emotional well-being. Mental health disorders such as anxiety, depression, and post-traumatic stress disorder (PTSD) are becoming increasingly prevalent in today's society. Energy medicine approaches, such as mindfulness-based practices, meditation, and breathwork, have been shown to reduce symptoms of anxiety and depression, improve mood, and enhance overall emotional resilience. These practices help individuals connect with their inner resources, manage stress, and cultivate a sense of calm and balance.

Integrating energy medicine with conventional cancer care is another promising avenue. Cancer treatments often come with side effects that impact a patient's overall well-being. Energy medicine modalities such as Reiki and therapeutic touch can provide support by reducing treatment-related anxiety and stress, improving quality of life, and supporting the body's healing processes. While energy medicine does not claim to cure cancer, it can be an invaluable addition to a comprehensive cancer care plan, providing comfort and enhancing the overall patient experience.

Energy medicine is also finding applications in the realm of preventive healthcare. Recognizing that imbalances in the energy systems can manifest as physical symptoms before the onset of disease, energy medicine techniques can be used to identify and address energetic imbalances at an early stage. By restoring balance and optimizing energy flow, individuals may be able to prevent the progression of certain conditions or maintain a state of well-being.

The integration of energy medicine into modern healthcare requires collaboration and open-mindedness among healthcare professionals. Many medical institutions are now offering integrative medicine programs that incorporate energy medicine techniques alongside conventional treatments. This allows patients to receive a comprehensive and individualized approach to their healthcare needs.

It is important to note that energy medicine should be practiced by qualified professionals who have received appropriate training and certification. Healthcare providers who integrate energy medicine into their practice undergo rigorous training to ensure safe and effective application of these modalities.

Chapter Two

The Human Energy System

The human body is a complex and remarkable organism that operates on intricate systems and processes. Beyond the physical structures and functions, there is an underlying energy system that plays a crucial role in maintaining health and well-being. Understanding the human energy system is fundamental to comprehending the principles and practices of energy medicine. Below we will explore the components and functions of the human energy system, shedding light on how it influences our physical, emotional, and spiritual states.

At the core of the human energy system are the energy centers, often referred to as chakras. Chakras are spinning wheels or vortexes of energy that are located along the body's midline. There are seven main chakras, each associated with different aspects of our being. Starting from the base of the spine and moving upwards, the chakras are the Root Chakra, Sacral Chakra, Solar Plexus Chakra, Heart Chakra, Throat Chakra, Third Eye Chakra, and Crown Chakra.

Each chakra is connected to specific physical organs, endocrine glands, and psychological functions. For example, the Root Chakra, located at the base of the spine, is associated with the sense of grounding, stability, and physical vitality. The Sacral Chakra, situated in the lower abdomen, is linked to emotions, creativity, and sexuality. The Crown Chakra, located at the top of the head, is associated with spiritual connection and higher consciousness.

The chakras are not only interconnected with each other but also with the body's energy pathways or meridians. Meridians are channels through which energy, often referred to as qi or prana, flows. These meridians form a complex network throughout the body, connecting the organs, tissues, and energy centers. The uninterrupted flow of energy along the meridians is essential for maintaining optimal health and well-being.

Another significant component of the human energy system is the aura. The aura is an electromagnetic energy field that surrounds the physical body. It is composed of multiple layers, each with its unique vibrational frequency. The aura interacts with the environment and other energy fields, providing information about a person's energetic state.

The aura reflects an individual's physical, emotional, mental, and spiritual well-being. It can be influenced by thoughts, emotions, and external factors. When the energy in the aura is balanced and harmonious, it contributes to overall health and vitality. However, imbalances or disturbances in the aura can manifest as physical symptoms or emotional and mental distress.

Energy medicine techniques aim to restore balance and optimize the flow of energy within the human energy system. Practitioners work with the chakras, meridians, and aura to identify and address any imbalances or blockages. Various modalities, such as acupuncture, Reiki, and sound healing, are used to promote the free flow of energy, release stagnant energy, and restore energetic harmony.

Acupuncture involves the insertion of thin needles into specific points along the meridians to restore the flow of energy. By stimulating these points, energy blockages can be cleared, and the body's natural healing mechanisms can be activated. Acupuncture has been shown to be effective in treating various conditions, including pain, digestive disorders, and emotional imbalances.

Reiki, on the other hand, is a hands-on healing technique that aims to channel universal life force energy to the recipient. The practitioner acts as a conduit, directing healing energy to the client's energy centers and aura. Reiki promotes deep relaxation, reduces stress, and supports the body's self-healing abilities. It is often used in conjunction with other medical treatments to enhance overall well-being.

Sound healing utilizes the vibrational frequencies of sound to influence the human energy system. Different sounds, such as singing

The energy body and its components

In the realm of energy medicine, the concept of the energy body forms the foundation of understanding and practice. It recognizes that beyond the physical body, there exists a complex system of energy that influences our health, emotions, and overall well-being. By exploring the components of the energy body, we can gain insight into the principles and practices of energy medicine. Below we will delve into the fascinating components of the energy body, shedding light on the aura, meridians, and energy vortices.

At the core of the energy body is the aura, an electromagnetic field that surrounds and interpenetrates the physical body. The aura is composed of multiple layers, each with its unique vibrational frequency and color. It acts as a subtle energy field that reflects and interacts with the individual's physical, emotional, mental, and spiritual states. The aura can extend several feet from the body and provides valuable information about a person's overall energetic well-being.

The aura is believed to be influenced by thoughts, emotions, and external factors, making it a dynamic and responsive field. When the energy in the aura is balanced and harmonious, it supports health and vitality. However, imbalances or disturbances in the aura can manifest as physical symptoms, emotional distress, or mental unease. Energy medicine techniques aim to restore balance and optimize the energy flow within the aura.

Meridians are another essential component of the energy body. These are channels through which energy, often referred to as qi or prana, flows. Meridians form a complex network throughout the body, connecting organs, tissues, and energy centers. There are twelve main meridians, each associated with specific organs and bodily functions. The meridians are responsible for the distribution of energy, ensuring that it reaches all parts of the body, nourishing and supporting its various systems.

Energy blockages or imbalances along the meridians can disrupt the flow of energy and contribute to physical or emotional discomfort. Acupuncture, a well-known energy medicine practice, involves the insertion of thin needles into specific points along the meridians to restore the flow of energy. By stimulating these points, energy blockages can be cleared, and the body's natural healing mechanisms can be activated.

In addition to the meridians, energy vortices known as chakras are key components of the energy body. Chakras are spinning wheels or vortexes of energy located at specific points along the body's midline. They correspond to different aspects of our being, such as physical vitality, emotions, creativity, intuition, and spiritual connection. There are seven main chakras, each associated with specific physical organs, endocrine glands, and psychological functions.

The chakras are interconnected with each other and influence the overall energetic state of an individual. When the chakras are balanced and functioning optimally, the energy flows smoothly throughout the energy body, supporting health and well-being. However, imbalances or blockages in the chakras can lead to physical or emotional disturbances. Energy medicine techniques focus on balancing and harmonizing the chakras to promote energetic alignment and enhance overall well-being.

The crown chakra, located at the top of the head, is associated with spiritual connection and higher consciousness. It is often depicted as a thousand-petaled lotus flower, symbolizing expanded awareness and enlightenment. The third-eye chakra, situated between the eyebrows, is associated with intuition, perception, and spiritual insight. The throat chakra governs communication, self-expression, and the ability to speak one's truth. The heart chakra is related to love, compassion, and emotional healing. The solar plexus chakra is associated with personal power, confidence, and self-esteem. The sacral chakra, located in the

Chakras and their functions

Chakras are energy centers within the human body that play a vital role in maintaining physical, emotional, and spiritual well-being. Stemming from ancient traditions, chakras are integral to the practice of energy medicine. Understanding the functions of each chakra can provide valuable insights into the principles and techniques used to balance and harmonize the body's energy. Below we will explore the seven main chakras, their locations, and their functions in relation to energy medicine.

The Root Chakra, or Muladhara, is located at the base of the spine. It is associated with our sense of stability, grounding, and physical vitality. This chakra governs our connection to the physical world, ensuring a solid foundation for our well-being. When the Root Chakra is balanced, we feel secure, confident, and able to handle life's challenges. Imbalances in this chakra can manifest as physical ailments, financial difficulties, or feelings of fear and insecurity. Energy medicine techniques can be used to restore balance and activate the Root Chakra, promoting a sense of stability and physical vitality.

Moving up the body, we come to the Sacral Chakra, or Svadhisthana, located in the lower abdomen. This chakra is associated with our emotions, creativity, and sexuality. It governs our ability to experience pleasure, embrace our desires, and express ourselves creatively. When the Sacral Chakra is balanced, we feel a sense of joy, passion, and emotional well-being. Imbalances in this chakra can lead to issues such as emotional instability, sexual difficulties, or a lack of creative inspiration. Energy medicine techniques can be used to stimulate and harmonize the Sacral Chakra, allowing for a free flow of emotional and creative energy.

The Solar Plexus Chakra, or Manipura, is located in the upper abdomen. It is often referred to as our power center, as it governs our sense of personal power, confidence, and self-esteem. This chakra is associated with our ability to assert ourselves, make decisions, and take action in the world. When the Solar Plexus Chakra is balanced, we feel a strong sense of self-worth, motivation, and empowerment. Imbalances in this chakra can manifest as low self-esteem, indecisiveness, or a lack of motivation. Energy medicine techniques can be used to activate and balance the Solar Plexus Chakra, fostering a sense of personal power and confidence.

Moving further up, we come to the Heart Chakra, or Anahata, located at the center of the chest. This chakra governs our ability to give and receive love, compassion, and forgiveness. It is associated with our connections with others, as well as our ability to connect with ourselves on a deep level. When the Heart Chakra is balanced, we experience love, compassion, and empathy towards ourselves and others. Imbalances in this chakra can lead to issues such as difficulty forming healthy relationships, a lack of self-love, or an inability to forgive. Energy medicine techniques can be used to open and balance the Heart Chakra, allowing for the free flow of love and compassion.

Moving up to the Throat Chakra, or Vishuddha, located at the base of the throat. This chakra governs our ability to communicate effectively, express ourselves authentically, and speak our truth. It is associated with clear and honest communication, both verbally and non-verbally. When the Throat Chakra is balanced, we can express ourselves clearly and confidently, and our communication with others is harmonious. Imbalances in this chakra can lead to issues such as difficulty expressing oneself, fear of public speaking, or frequent misunderstandings in communication. Energy medicine techniques can be used to balance

Meridians and energy pathways

Within the realm of energy medicine, the concept of meridians and energy pathways forms a fundamental aspect of understanding and working with the body's energy system. These channels, through which energy flows, are vital to maintaining health and well-being. By exploring the nature of meridians and energy pathways, we can gain insight into the principles and practices of energy medicine. Below we will delve into the fascinating world of meridians and energy pathways, their functions, and their significance in relation to energy medicine.

Meridians are pathways through which vital energy, known as qi or prana, flows throughout the body. These energy pathways connect various organs, tissues, and systems, forming an intricate network. The concept of meridians originated in ancient Chinese medicine and has been used for thousands of years to diagnose and treat illnesses.

There are twelve main meridians in the body, each associated with a specific organ or organ system. These meridians run bilaterally, meaning they exist on both sides of the body. They are classified into six yin meridians, which are more inward and nourishing, and six yang meridians, which are more outward and active.

The meridians are named according to the organ they are associated with. For example, the Lung Meridian runs from the chest to the thumb and is responsible for the circulation of qi in the lungs. The Stomach Meridian runs from the face to the second toe and governs the digestion and assimilation of food. Each meridian has a specific pathway and a unique flow of energy that corresponds to its associated organ or organ system.

The flow of energy within the meridians is not static but rather dynamic. It is influenced by various factors such as time of day, seasons, emotions, and lifestyle. When the flow of energy within the meridians is smooth and balanced, health and well-being are maintained. However, if there are blockages or imbalances in the energy flow, it can lead to physical or emotional disharmony.

Energy medicine techniques, such as acupuncture and acupressure, work with the meridians to restore the balance and flow of energy. Acupuncture involves the insertion of thin needles into specific points along the meridians to stimulate and regulate the energy flow. Acupressure, on the other hand, applies pressure to these points using the hands, fingers, or specific tools. Both techniques aim to clear blockages, promote the smooth flow of energy, and activate the body's natural healing abilities.

In addition to the twelve main meridians, there are also smaller energy pathways or microsystems within the body. These microsystems, such as the ear, hand, and foot, contain reflex points that correspond to various organs and systems. Stimulating these points can have a therapeutic effect on the corresponding areas of the body. For example, in ear acupuncture, specific points on the ear are stimulated to address health issues throughout the body.

The concept of energy pathways extends beyond the physical body to include the energy field surrounding and interpenetrating it. This field, often referred to as the biofield or aura, is composed of electromagnetic energy and subtle vibrations. It interacts with the physical body and serves as a template for its functioning.

The biofield contains its own network of energy pathways, often referred to as energy channels or nadis. These channels are similar to meridians but operate on a more subtle level. They facilitate the flow of energy within the biofield and influence the physical, emotional, and spiritual aspects of an individual.

Energy medicine techniques, such as Reiki and pranic healing, work with the biofield and its energy pathways to restore balance and harmony. Reiki practitioners, for example, act as

The aura and its significance

In the realm of energy medicine, the concept of the aura holds great significance. The aura is an electromagnetic energy field that surrounds and interpenetrates the human body. It is an essential component of the energy system and plays a crucial role in our physical, emotional, and spiritual well-being. Understanding the nature and significance of the aura is key to comprehending the principles and practices of energy medicine. Below we will explore the aura, its composition, functions, and its significance in relation to energy medicine.

The aura is often described as a luminous field that emanates from the body, extending several feet in all directions. It is composed of multiple layers, each with its own unique vibrational frequency and color. These layers interact and blend to create a dynamic energy field that reflects and interacts with our physical, emotional, mental, and spiritual states.

The aura serves as a subtle energetic blueprint of the individual, providing valuable information about their overall energetic well-being. It is sensitive to thoughts, emotions, and external factors, making it a responsive and dynamic field. Changes in our thoughts and emotions can influence the aura, and conversely, imbalances or disturbances in the aura can impact our physical and emotional states.

One significant function of the aura is to act as a protective barrier, shielding us from external influences and energies. It acts as an energetic filter, allowing in energies that are beneficial and supportive while repelling those that are detrimental or disharmonious. When the aura is strong and vibrant, it enhances our resilience and protects us from energetic imbalances or intrusions.

The aura also serves as a vehicle for communication and interaction with the world around us. It interacts with the auras of other individuals, animals, and the environment, allowing for subtle exchanges of energy and information. This energetic communication influences our relationships and interactions with others, as well as our overall sense of connection and belonging.

Energy medicine techniques focus on working with the aura to restore balance and promote well-being. Practitioners use various modalities to assess the aura's condition and address any imbalances or disturbances. These techniques aim to clear stagnant or congested energy, repair any energetic leaks or holes, and harmonize the aura's layers. By optimizing the health and vibrancy of the aura, energy medicine promotes overall physical, emotional, and spiritual well-being.

The colors of the aura are an essential aspect of its significance. Each layer of the aura is associated with specific colors, which can provide insight into a person's energetic state and overall well-being. For example, a vibrant and balanced aura may exhibit bright and radiant colors, indicating good health, vitality, and positive emotions. On the other hand, a dull or muddy aura may indicate energetic imbalances or emotional distress.

Energy medicine practitioners are trained to perceive and interpret the colors of the aura to gain a deeper understanding of an individual's energetic state. They can identify areas of congestion, depletion, or imbalance and tailor their energy healing techniques accordingly. By addressing specific colors or energetic patterns within the aura, practitioners can restore balance and promote healing on multiple levels.

The significance of the aura extends beyond its individual-level impact to collective consciousness and the interconnectedness of all beings. The aura represents our interconnectedness with others, as it interacts with and blends with the auras of those around us. This energetic interplay contributes to the overall energetic field of a group or community.

Energy medicine techniques, such as group healing or collective meditation, harness the power of the collective aura to promote healing and transformation. By coming together with shared intention and focus, individuals can create a collective energetic field that supports individual and collective well-being.

Chapter Three

Energy Medicine Techniques

Energy medicine encompasses a wide range of techniques and modalities that aim to restore balance and promote healing in the body's energy system. These techniques have been used for centuries in various cultures around the world and have gained recognition in modern healthcare settings. Below we will explore some of the most common energy medicine techniques, shedding light on their principles, applications, and benefits.

Acupuncture is a well-known energy medicine technique originating from ancient Chinese medicine. It involves the insertion of thin needles into specific points along the body's energy pathways, known as meridians. By stimulating these points, acupuncture aims to restore the smooth flow of energy, clear blockages, and promote the body's natural healing processes. Acupuncture has been shown to be effective in managing pain, reducing inflammation, and addressing a wide range of physical and emotional conditions.

Reiki is a Japanese healing technique that utilizes the transfer of universal life force energy through the practitioner's hands to the recipient. The practitioner acts as a channel, allowing healing energy to flow into the recipient's energy field. Reiki promotes deep relaxation, stress reduction, and overall well-being. It can be used to address physical ailments, emotional imbalances, and spiritual distress. Reiki is often used as a complementary therapy alongside conventional medical treatments to enhance the healing process.

Therapeutic Touch is a hands-on healing technique that involves the practitioner placing their hands near the recipient's body to detect and balance energy imbalances. The practitioner uses their hands to assess the recipient's energy field and then uses gentle touch or sweeping motions to clear blockages and restore harmony. Therapeutic Touch has been shown to reduce pain, anxiety, and stress, and promote relaxation and wound healing.

Sound healing is a technique that utilizes the vibrational frequencies of sound to influence the body's energy field. Different sounds, such as vocal toning, singing bowls, or tuning forks, are used to create harmonious vibrations that interact with the energy system. Sound healing can help release stagnant energy, promote relaxation, and balance the chakras. It has been used to support emotional healing, enhance meditation practices, and promote overall well-being.

Crystal therapy involves the use of crystals and gemstones to balance and harmonize the body's energy. Crystals are believed to possess unique vibrational properties that interact with the energy field, promoting healing and well-being. Practitioners place crystals on or around the body's energy centers or incorporate them into jewelry. Each crystal is associated with different healing properties, and specific crystals are selected based on the individual's needs. Crystal therapy can be used to address physical ailments, emotional imbalances, and spiritual growth.

Meditation is a practice that cultivates deep relaxation, focused awareness, and connection with the inner self. It can be used as a standalone energy medicine technique or as a complementary practice alongside other modalities. Meditation helps quiet the mind, reduce stress, and enhance self-awareness. It promotes the balance and flow of energy within the body, allowing for healing and restoration.

Breathwork involves conscious breathing techniques that facilitate the release of stagnant energy and the activation of the body's natural healing processes. By focusing on deep, rhythmic breathing, individuals can increase oxygen flow, clear energetic blockages, and promote a sense of calm and balance. Breathwork is often used to support stress reduction, emotional healing, and spiritual exploration.

These are just a few examples of the many energy medicine techniques available. It is important to note that energy medicine is not meant to replace conventional medical care but rather to complement it. It can be used alongside other treatments to enhance overall well-being and support the body's natural healing abilities.

Acupuncture and acupressure

Acupuncture and acupressure are two ancient healing techniques that have been used for centuries in various cultures around the world. Stemming from traditional Chinese medicine, these practices are based on the concept of energy flow within the body and its impact on health and well-being. In the realm of energy medicine, acupuncture and acupressure are powerful tools for restoring balance and promoting healing. Below we will explore the principles, applications, and benefits of acupuncture and acupressure in relation to energy medicine.

Acupuncture is a technique that involves the insertion of thin needles into specific points along the body's energy pathways, known as meridians. According to traditional Chinese medicine, the body is permeated by a complex network of meridians through which vital energy, known as qi, flows. The uninterrupted flow of qi is essential for maintaining health and well-being, and any blockages or imbalances in the meridians can lead to physical or emotional disturbances.

By inserting needles into specific acupuncture points along the meridians, an acupuncturist aims to restore the smooth flow of qi, clear blockages, and promote the body's natural healing processes. The needles are usually left in place for a certain period, during which the recipient may experience sensations such as tingling, warmth, or a sense of heaviness. These sensations are believed to be indications of the movement of qi within the body.

Acupuncture has been shown to be effective in managing pain, reducing inflammation, and addressing a wide range of physical and emotional conditions. It is commonly used to alleviate musculoskeletal pain, such as back pain, joint pain, and headaches. Acupuncture can also be beneficial for digestive disorders, respiratory conditions, hormonal imbalances, and mental health conditions such as anxiety and depression. By restoring the balance and flow of qi, acupuncture promotes the body's self-healing abilities and supports overall well-being.

Acupressure is a technique that is similar to acupuncture but does not involve the use of needles. Instead, it applies pressure to specific acupuncture points using the hands, fingers, or specific tools. The pressure can be applied through various techniques, such as rubbing, tapping, or kneading. Like acupuncture, acupressure aims to restore the flow of qi and promote balance within the body's energy system.

Acupressure can be easily practiced by individuals on themselves or by trained practitioners on others. It is a versatile technique that can be applied in various settings, such as hospitals, clinics, or even self-care routines at home. Acupressure is often used as a complementary therapy alongside other medical treatments to enhance their effectiveness and promote overall well-being.

Both acupuncture and acupressure work on the same principles of restoring balance and promoting the flow of energy within the body. They are based on the concept of meridians and acupuncture points, which are specific locations along the meridians where the energy flow can be accessed and influenced.

The effectiveness of acupuncture and acupressure has been supported by scientific research, which has shown their ability to stimulate the release of endorphins, the body's natural pain-relieving chemicals. These techniques have also been found to modulate the autonomic nervous system, reduce inflammation, and promote relaxation and stress reduction.

Furthermore, acupuncture and acupressure are not limited to physical ailments but also address emotional and mental imbalances. They can help reduce anxiety, improve sleep, and enhance overall emotional well-being. By promoting the balance and flow of energy, these techniques support the mind-body connection and contribute to holistic healing.

It is important to note that acupuncture and acupressure should be practiced by qualified professionals who have received appropriate training and certification. They should be tailored to

Reiki and healing touch

Reiki and Healing Touch are two popular healing modalities that operate within the realm of energy medicine. Both techniques involve the channeling of universal life force energy to promote healing and restore balance within the body's energy system. Rooted in ancient wisdom and spiritual practices, Reiki and Healing Touch have gained recognition and acceptance in modern healthcare settings. Below we will explore the principles, applications, and benefits of Reiki and Healing Touch in relation to energy medicine.

Reiki, originating from Japan, is a healing technique that utilizes the transfer of universal life force energy through the practitioner's hands to the recipient. The word "Reiki" can be translated as "universal life energy" or "spiritually guided life force energy." It is based on the belief that energy flows through all living beings, and disruptions or imbalances in this energy can lead to physical, emotional, and spiritual ailments.

During a Reiki session, the practitioner acts as a channel for healing energy, directing it to the recipient's energy field. The practitioner's hands are placed gently on or near specific areas of the body, allowing the energy to flow where it is needed most. The recipient may experience sensations such as warmth, tingling, or deep relaxation during the session.

Reiki is a non-invasive technique that aims to promote relaxation, reduce stress, and support the body's natural healing processes. It is often used as a complementary therapy alongside conventional medical treatments to enhance overall well-being. Reiki can be beneficial for various physical conditions, including chronic pain, fatigue, and immune system disorders. It can also help address emotional imbalances, promote mental clarity, and facilitate spiritual growth.

Healing Touch, on the other hand, is a healing modality that utilizes touch to influence the body's energy field and promote healing. It is a contemporary approach to energy healing that draws from various traditions, including ancient healing practices and modern scientific knowledge. Healing Touch practitioners use their hands to detect and balance energy imbalances within the recipient's energy field.

During a Healing Touch session, the practitioner assesses the recipient's energy field and uses gentle touch or sweeping motions to clear blockages and restore harmony. The goal is to create a state of deep relaxation and support the body's natural ability to heal itself. Healing Touch has been found to reduce pain, anxiety, and stress, and promote wound healing.

Both Reiki and Healing Touch are based on the belief that the body has an innate ability to heal itself, and that by facilitating the flow of healing energy, this natural healing process can be enhanced. These techniques recognize the interconnectedness of the physical, emotional, mental, and spiritual aspects of an individual and aim to address imbalances on all levels.

The effectiveness of Reiki and Healing Touch has been supported by anecdotal evidence and growing scientific research. Studies have shown that these techniques can reduce pain, anxiety, and depression, and enhance overall well-being. They have been used successfully in various healthcare settings, including hospitals, clinics, and hospice care.

One of the key benefits of Reiki and Healing Touch is their ability to induce a state of deep relaxation and reduce stress. Stress is a contributing factor to many physical and emotional ailments, and by promoting relaxation, these techniques support the body's self-healing mechanisms. The relaxation response triggered by Reiki and Healing Touch can have a positive impact on blood pressure, heart rate, and immune function.

Another significant benefit of Reiki and Healing Touch is their non-invasive nature. They do not involve the use of medications, procedures, or invasive techniques, making them safe and accessible to people of all ages and conditions. These techniques can be used alongside conventional medical treatments and have no known adverse effects.

It is important to note that Re

Chapter Four

Qi Gong and Tai Chi

Qi Gong and Tai Chi are ancient Chinese practices that have been utilized for centuries to promote health, vitality, and spiritual well-being. Rooted in traditional Chinese medicine, these practices are grounded in the concept of energy flow within the body and its impact on overall health. In the realm of energy medicine, Qi Gong and Tai Chi are regarded as powerful tools for restoring balance and harmonizing the body's energy system. Below we will explore the principles, applications, and benefits of Qi Gong and Tai Chi in relation to energy medicine.

Qi Gong, which translates to "cultivation of vital energy," is a holistic system that combines movement, breathwork, meditation, and intention to cultivate and balance the body's energy. It is based on the belief that vital energy, known as qi, flows through the body along energy pathways called meridians. Qi Gong practices are designed to promote the smooth flow of qi, clear blockages, and enhance the body's self-healing abilities.

Qi Gong exercises vary in their forms, but all involve gentle movements, deep breathing, and focused intention. The slow and deliberate movements are designed to stimulate the flow of qi, increase flexibility, and enhance physical and mental well-being. Through regular practice, individuals can cultivate a heightened sense of energy, reduce stress, and promote a state of relaxation and inner peace.

Qi Gong can be beneficial for a wide range of physical and emotional conditions. It has been found to support cardiovascular health, improve balance and coordination, strengthen the immune system, and reduce chronic pain. Qi Gong also has a positive impact on mental and emotional well-being by reducing stress, anxiety, and depression.

Tai Chi, also known as Tai Chi Chuan, is a martial art form that originated in ancient China. It is characterized by slow, flowing movements, deep breathing, and mindful awareness. Like Qi Gong, Tai Chi is rooted in the principles of balancing and harmonizing the body's energy.

Tai Chi incorporates elements of martial arts, philosophy, and meditation. Its movements are fluid, continuous, and graceful, resembling a slow-motion dance. The focus is on maintaining a relaxed and centered state while moving through a series of postures and transitions.

Tai Chi is known for its many health benefits. It enhances balance and stability, improves posture and body alignment, and strengthens the muscles and joints. Regular practice of Tai Chi has been shown to reduce blood pressure, improve cardiovascular health, and enhance overall physical fitness. Additionally, Tai Chi promotes mental clarity, concentration, and emotional well-being.

Both Qi Gong and Tai Chi have profound effects on the body's energy system. They facilitate the flow of qi, stimulate energy points and meridians, and balance the yin and yang energies within the body. These practices harmonize the body, mind, and spirit, fostering a sense of unity and holistic well-being.

One of the unique aspects of Qi Gong and Tai Chi is their focus on mindful awareness and intention. Practitioners are encouraged to cultivate a state of present-moment awareness, directing their attention to the body's movements, sensations, and breath. This mindful approach deepens the connection between the mind and body, amplifying the therapeutic effects of these practices.

Moreover, Qi Gong and Tai Chi promote deep diaphragmatic breathing, which has a calming and grounding effect on the nervous system. By emphasizing slow, rhythmic breathwork, these practices activate the body's relaxation response, reduce stress, and enhance overall resilience.

Another significant aspect of Qi Gong and Tai Chi is their accessibility. These practices are suitable for people of all ages and physical abilities. They can be modified to accommodate individual needs, making them accessible to those with physical limitations or health conditions. Qi Gong and Tai Chi can be practiced in various settings, including

Therapeutic touch and energy manipulation

Therapeutic Touch and energy manipulation are practices that focus on working with subtle energy fields to promote healing and well-being. Rooted in the principles of energy medicine, these techniques recognize the vital role of energy in maintaining health and balance. Therapeutic Touch and energy manipulation offer non-invasive approaches to accessing and manipulating the body's energy, facilitating the body's natural healing processes. Below we will explore the principles, applications, and benefits of Therapeutic Touch and energy manipulation in relation to energy medicine.

Therapeutic Touch is a healing technique that involves the practitioner using their hands to detect and balance the recipient's energy field. It is based on the understanding that every individual has an energy field that extends beyond the physical body. By assessing the recipient's energy field, the practitioner can identify areas of imbalance or energetic congestion.

During a Therapeutic Touch session, the practitioner uses their hands to clear blockages, restore balance, and promote the flow of energy within the recipient's energy field. This is achieved through gentle touch or by working within the energy field without physical contact. The practitioner's intention and focused attention play a crucial role in directing the healing energy to the recipient.

Therapeutic Touch can be effective in reducing pain, anxiety, and stress, and promoting relaxation and well-being. It is often used in healthcare settings as a complementary therapy alongside conventional medical treatments. Therapeutic Touch can be applied to various conditions, including acute and chronic pain, surgical recovery, and emotional distress. By working with the energy field, Therapeutic Touch facilitates the body's natural healing processes and supports overall health.

Energy manipulation techniques encompass a variety of approaches aimed at manipulating the body's energy field. These techniques involve directing or manipulating the energy flow to restore balance, remove blockages, and promote healing. Energy manipulation can be performed with or without physical touch, depending on the practitioner's modality and the needs of the recipient.

One well-known energy manipulation technique is polarity therapy, which combines gentle touch, energetic bodywork, and verbal counseling. Polarity therapy focuses on balancing the body's energy flow by working with energy centers, known as chakras, and energy pathways, known as meridians. By assessing and balancing the energetic patterns within the body, polarity therapy aims to restore harmony and support overall well-being.

Craniosacral therapy is another energy manipulation technique that focuses on the subtle rhythms and movements of the cerebrospinal fluid. Practitioners use gentle touch to assess and enhance the flow of this fluid, which is believed to influence the health and functioning of the central nervous system. Craniosacral therapy aims to release restrictions and promote balance within the craniosacral system, thereby supporting the body's self-healing abilities.

The benefits of energy manipulation techniques are similar to those of Therapeutic Touch. These techniques can promote relaxation, reduce pain and stress, enhance the body's natural healing processes, and support overall well-being. By working with the body's energy field, energy manipulation techniques aim to restore balance and harmony on multiple levels, addressing the physical, emotional, and spiritual aspects of an individual.

The effectiveness of Therapeutic Touch and energy manipulation techniques has been supported by research and clinical experience. Although the mechanisms by which these techniques work are still not fully understood, studies have shown their positive impact on various conditions, including pain management, anxiety reduction, wound healing, and symptom relief.

One theory is that Therapeutic Touch and energy manipulation techniques influence the body's biofield, a complex matrix of electromagnetic and subtle energies that interpenetrates and surrounds the physical body. By manipulating the biofield, these techniques can influence the flow of energy and information within the body, promoting balance and supporting healing.

It is important to note

Energy Medicine Modalities

1. Energy Medicine Modalities: Exploring the Diversity of Healing Techniques

Energy medicine encompasses a wide range of modalities and techniques that aim to restore balance, promote healing, and enhance overall well-being. These modalities work with the body's energy system, recognizing the vital role of energy in maintaining health and harmony. From ancient practices to contemporary approaches, energy medicine offers a diverse array of techniques. Below we will explore some of the most commonly used energy medicine modalities, highlighting their principles, applications, and benefits.

2. Acupuncture: Acupuncture is a traditional Chinese medicine practice that involves the insertion of thin needles into specific points along the body's energy pathways, known as meridians. By stimulating these points, acupuncture aims to restore the smooth flow of energy, clear blockages, and promote the body's natural healing processes. Acupuncture has been shown to be effective in managing pain, reducing inflammation, and addressing a wide range of physical and emotional conditions.

3. Reiki: Reiki is a Japanese healing technique that utilizes the transfer of universal life force energy through the practitioner's hands to the recipient. The practitioner acts as a channel, allowing healing energy to flow into the recipient's energy field. Reiki promotes deep relaxation, stress reduction, and overall well-being. It can be used to address physical ailments, emotional imbalances, and spiritual distress. Reiki is often used as a complementary therapy alongside conventional medical treatments to enhance the healing process.

4. Therapeutic Touch: Therapeutic Touch is a hands-on healing technique that involves the practitioner placing their hands near the recipient's body to detect and balance energy imbalances. The practitioner uses their hands to assess the recipient's energy field and then uses gentle touch or sweeping motions to clear blockages and restore harmony. Therapeutic Touch has been shown to reduce pain, anxiety, and stress, and promote relaxation and wound healing.

5. Crystal Therapy: Crystal therapy involves the use of crystals and gemstones to balance and harmonize the body's energy. Crystals are believed to possess unique vibrational properties that interact with the energy field, promoting healing and well-being. Practitioners place crystals on or around the body's energy centers or incorporate them into jewelry. Each crystal is associated with different healing properties, and specific crystals are selected based on the individual's needs. Crystal therapy can be used to address physical ailments, emotional imbalances, and spiritual growth.

6. Sound Healing: Sound healing utilizes the vibrational frequencies of sound to influence the body's energy field. Different sounds, such as vocal toning, singing bowls, or tuning forks, are used to create harmonious vibrations that interact with the energy system. Sound healing can help release stagnant energy, promote relaxation, and balance the chakras. It has been used to support emotional healing, enhance meditation practices, and promote overall well-being.

7. Qi Gong and Tai Chi: Qi Gong and Tai Chi are ancient Chinese practices that combine movement, breathwork, and meditation to cultivate and balance the body's energy. Qi Gong involves gentle movements, deep breathing, and focused intention to promote the smooth flow of qi and enhance well-being. Tai Chi incorporates slow, flowing movements and mindful awareness to harmonize the body, mind, and spirit. Both practices have been found to reduce stress, improve balance and coordination, and enhance overall physical and mental well-being.

8. Craniosacral Therapy: Craniosacral therapy focuses on the subtle rhythms and movements of the cerebrospinal fluid to influence the health and functioning of the central nervous system. Practitioners use gentle touch to assess and enhance the flow of this fluid, aiming to release restrictions and promote balance within the craniosacral system. Craniosacral

therapy has been shown to reduce pain, support relaxation, and facilitate the body's

Biofeedback and neurofeedback

Biofeedback and neurofeedback are innovative approaches within the realm of energy medicine that focus on the mind-body connection and the ability to influence physiological processes through awareness and self-regulation. These modalities utilize advanced technology to provide real-time feedback on various physiological parameters, allowing individuals to gain insight and control over their own bodily functions. Below we will explore the principles, applications, and benefits of biofeedback and neurofeedback in relation to energy medicine.

Biofeedback is a technique that involves monitoring and measuring physiological functions, such as heart rate, blood pressure, muscle tension, and skin conductance, and providing real-time feedback to the individual. This feedback is typically visual or auditory, enabling individuals to observe and learn to control their physiological responses. By increasing awareness and developing self-regulation skills, individuals can modify their body's responses to stressors and promote overall well-being.

The process of biofeedback involves attaching sensors to the body to monitor specific physiological signals. The data collected by these sensors is then processed by a computer, which provides feedback in the form of visual cues, sounds, or even virtual reality simulations. Through this feedback, individuals can learn to recognize patterns and make conscious changes to their physiological responses.

Biofeedback techniques have been used in various clinical and non-clinical settings to address a wide range of conditions, including stress-related disorders, chronic pain, anxiety, and migraines. By learning to regulate their physiological responses, individuals can reduce symptoms, enhance relaxation, and improve their overall quality of life.

Neurofeedback, a subset of biofeedback, specifically focuses on monitoring and providing feedback on brainwave activity. It involves the use of an electroencephalogram (EEG) to measure the electrical activity of the brain. The individual's brainwave patterns are then translated into visual or auditory feedback, allowing them to observe and learn to modulate their brain activity.

Neurofeedback training aims to promote optimal brain function by teaching individuals to self-regulate their brainwave patterns. By guiding the brain into desired states, such as increased focus, relaxation, or reduced anxiety, individuals can improve cognitive performance, emotional well-being, and overall mental health.

Neurofeedback has been utilized in various settings, including clinical practice, sports performance, and personal development. It has shown promising results in addressing attention deficit hyperactivity disorder (ADHD), anxiety disorders, insomnia, and even traumatic brain injuries. By training the brain to function more efficiently, neurofeedback empowers individuals to enhance their mental and emotional states.

Both biofeedback and neurofeedback operate on the principle that the mind and body are interconnected, and individuals have the capacity to influence their physiological responses through awareness and self-regulation. These modalities provide individuals with valuable information about their own bodily functions, allowing them to make conscious changes that promote health and well-being.

The success of biofeedback and neurofeedback lies in their ability to tap into the body's innate self-regulatory mechanisms. By providing real-time feedback, individuals gain immediate information about the impact of their thoughts, emotions, and behaviors on their physiological responses. This heightened awareness allows them to develop self-control and make targeted adjustments to their body's reactions.

Moreover, biofeedback and neurofeedback techniques are non-invasive and drug-free, making them safe and accessible options for individuals seeking self-improvement and well-being. These modalities empower individuals to take an active role in their own health and provide them with tools to manage stress, improve performance, and enhance overall functioning.

Polarity therapy

Polarity therapy is a holistic healing modality that focuses on balancing the body's energy field to promote physical, emotional, and spiritual well-being. Developed by Dr. Randolph Stone, a chiropractor and osteopath, polarity therapy combines elements of Eastern and Western healing traditions to address energetic imbalances and enhance the body's natural healing abilities. Below we will explore the principles, applications, and benefits of polarity therapy in relation to energy medicine.

At the core of polarity therapy is the belief that energy flows through the body in specific patterns and that disruptions or blockages in this energy flow can lead to physical or emotional ailments. The practitioner of polarity therapy works with the body's energy system, including the electromagnetic field, energy centers (chakras), and energy pathways (meridians), to restore balance and harmony.

Polarity therapy sessions typically involve a combination of touch, movement, counseling, and energetic techniques. The practitioner assesses the client's energy field by gently scanning and palpating various points on the body. By identifying areas of energy congestion or depletion, the practitioner tailors the session to address specific imbalances.

One of the key techniques used in polarity therapy is energetic bodywork. The practitioner applies gentle touch and manipulations to specific points on the body to release energy blockages and restore the flow of energy. This touch can be light or deep, depending on the individual's needs and preferences. The goal is to activate the body's self-healing mechanisms and promote overall balance.

Another important aspect of polarity therapy is the recognition of the relationship between the physical body, emotions, and thoughts. The practitioner may engage in counseling or dialogue to help the client explore emotional patterns and belief systems that may contribute to energetic imbalances. By addressing these underlying factors, polarity therapy aims to support holistic healing and personal growth.

Polarity therapy is used to address a wide range of physical, emotional, and spiritual conditions. It can be effective in relieving musculoskeletal pain, reducing stress and anxiety, promoting relaxation, and supporting overall well-being. Polarity therapy has also been used as a complementary therapy for chronic conditions, such as fibromyalgia and digestive disorders.

One of the unique aspects of polarity therapy is its focus on the energetic patterns within the body. The practitioner recognizes that energy flows in a specific polarity, including positive, negative, and neutral charges. By balancing these polarities, polarity therapy aims to restore harmony and promote the body's natural ability to heal.

Polarity therapy also emphasizes the role of the breath in balancing and energizing the body. Breathing exercises and awareness techniques are often incorporated into sessions to support the flow of energy and enhance relaxation. Deep, conscious breathing is believed to facilitate the release of stagnant energy and promote overall vitality.

Additionally, polarity therapy recognizes the interconnectedness of the physical, emotional, and spiritual aspects of an individual. It aims to support the integration of these dimensions to achieve optimal well-being. By working with the body's energy field, polarity therapy provides a holistic framework for healing and personal growth.

It is important to note that polarity therapy is generally considered safe and non-invasive. It can be used as a standalone therapy or as a complement to other conventional or alternative treatments. However, it is essential to seek a qualified and trained polarity therapy practitioner to ensure safe and effective sessions.

Electromagnetic field therapy

Electromagnetic Field (EMF) therapy is a fascinating modality within the realm of energy medicine that utilizes electromagnetic fields to promote healing and overall well-being. It is based on the principle that electromagnetic energy plays a vital role in the body's functioning and that disturbances in this energy can lead to imbalances and health issues. Below we will explore the principles, applications, and benefits of electromagnetic field therapy in relation to energy medicine.

At the core of electromagnetic field therapy is the understanding that every cell in the body produces and responds to electromagnetic signals. These signals are essential for various physiological processes, including cellular communication, tissue repair, and overall cellular health. When there is a disruption or imbalance in these electromagnetic signals, it can lead to cellular dysfunction and contribute to the development of disease.

Electromagnetic field therapy involves the application of specific frequencies and intensities of electromagnetic fields to the body. This can be achieved through various methods, such as pulsed electromagnetic field therapy (PEMF), magnetic field therapy, or low-level laser therapy. These therapies aim to restore balance and optimize the body's natural electromagnetic energy.

Pulsed electromagnetic field therapy, in particular, has gained attention for its potential health benefits. This therapy utilizes electromagnetic fields that are delivered in brief pulses or frequencies. These pulses can penetrate deep into the body, reaching cells and tissues to promote healing and cellular regeneration.

Electromagnetic field therapy has been used to address a wide range of health conditions. It has shown promising results in promoting bone healing, reducing pain and inflammation, accelerating wound healing, and enhancing tissue repair. It has also been used to support mental health conditions, such as depression and anxiety, by stimulating brainwave activity and promoting relaxation.

One of the underlying mechanisms of electromagnetic field therapy is its influence on the body's bioelectric and electromagnetic systems. By providing external electromagnetic signals, this therapy can help restore balance and enhance cellular communication. It is believed that electromagnetic fields can modulate ion channels, influence cellular metabolism, and promote the release of growth factors, all of which contribute to cellular health and healing.

Furthermore, electromagnetic field therapy can have a positive impact on the body's energetic field. The energy field, often referred to as the biofield or aura, is an electromagnetic field that surrounds and permeates the body. By restoring balance and coherence to the body's electromagnetic field, electromagnetic field therapy can support the overall balance and flow of energy within the body.

Electromagnetic field therapy is non-invasive and generally well-tolerated. It can be used as a standalone therapy or in conjunction with other conventional or complementary treatments. However, it is important to note that electromagnetic field therapy may not be suitable for individuals with certain medical conditions or those with implanted electronic devices. It is always advisable to consult with a qualified healthcare practitioner before starting any new therapy.

It is important to distinguish between therapeutic electromagnetic fields used in electromagnetic field therapy and electromagnetic fields generated by electronic devices, such as cell phones or Wi-Fi signals. The therapeutic electromagnetic fields used in therapy are specifically designed and controlled to produce desired physiological effects, while excessive exposure to electronic device emissions may have different implications.

Craniosacral therapy

Craniosacral therapy is a gentle and non-invasive healing modality that focuses on the subtle rhythms and movements of the cerebrospinal fluid and their impact on the overall health of the body. Rooted in the principles of energy medicine, craniosacral therapy recognizes the interconnectedness of the physical, emotional, and energetic aspects of an individual. Below we will explore the principles, applications, and benefits of craniosacral therapy in relation to energy medicine.

At the core of craniosacral therapy is the concept that the body is imbued with a rhythmic pulsation known as the craniosacral rhythm. This rhythm arises from the subtle movement of cerebrospinal fluid, which bathes and nourishes the brain and spinal cord. Practitioners of craniosacral therapy use their hands to assess and manipulate this rhythm, facilitating its optimal expression and addressing any imbalances or restrictions.

During a craniosacral therapy session, the practitioner applies gentle touch and manipulation to specific areas of the body, including the cranium, spine, and sacrum. Through skilled palpation, the practitioner detects areas of tension, restriction, or stagnation within the craniosacral system. Using subtle movements and precise pressure, the practitioner works to release these restrictions and restore the natural flow and balance of cerebrospinal fluid.

Craniosacral therapy aims to promote the body's inherent self-healing mechanisms and support overall well-being. By enhancing the flow of cerebrospinal fluid, this therapy can have a positive impact on various physiological systems, including the nervous system, immune system, and musculoskeletal system.

One of the primary benefits of craniosacral therapy is its ability to reduce pain and tension. By releasing restrictions within the craniosacral system, this therapy can alleviate headaches, migraines, temporomandibular joint (TMJ) disorders, and other chronic pain conditions. It can also improve the function and mobility of the musculoskeletal system, promoting relaxation and flexibility.

Craniosacral therapy has been found to have a profound impact on the nervous system. It can support the regulation of the autonomic nervous system, reducing the effects of stress and promoting a state of deep relaxation. This therapy is often used to address conditions such as anxiety, insomnia, and post-traumatic stress disorder (PTSD), as it helps to calm the nervous system and restore balance.

Furthermore, craniosacral therapy recognizes the energetic aspects of the body and their influence on health and well-being. Practitioners of craniosacral therapy often work with the body's energy field and the energetic patterns within the craniosacral system. By balancing and harmonizing these energetic aspects, craniosacral therapy supports the overall flow of energy and contributes to holistic healing.

Craniosacral therapy is a versatile modality that can be applied to individuals of all ages, from newborns to the elderly. It has been used in various healthcare settings, including hospitals, clinics, and private practices. Craniosacral therapy can be integrated with other complementary therapies and conventional medical treatments to enhance their effectiveness and promote holistic well-being.

It is important to note that craniosacral therapy should be performed by qualified practitioners who have received appropriate training and certification. The practitioner's sensitivity, skill, and ability to establish a therapeutic relationship with the client are crucial aspects of a successful craniosacral therapy session.

Chapter Five

Energy Medicine and Emotional Healing

Energy medicine recognizes the intricate connection between the body, mind, and emotions, understanding that imbalances within the energy system can contribute to emotional distress and affect overall well-being. In recent years, there has been a growing appreciation for the role of energy medicine in supporting emotional healing and promoting inner harmony. Below we will explore the principles, techniques, and benefits of energy medicine in relation to emotional healing.

At the heart of energy medicine is the understanding that the body is composed of not just physical matter but also subtle energy fields. These energy fields, often referred to as the biofield or aura, interpenetrate and surround the physical body. They are believed to contain information and influence the overall health and well-being of an individual.

Emotions, too, are considered energetic in nature. Each emotion carries its own unique energetic frequency, and when emotions become imbalanced or suppressed, they can disrupt the flow of energy within the body. This energetic disturbance can contribute to physical discomfort, mental distress, and emotional imbalances.

Energy medicine techniques offer various approaches to address emotional healing and restore energetic balance. Here are some commonly used techniques:

2. Energetic Clearing: Energetic clearing techniques aim to release stagnant or negative energy from the energy field. These techniques can include smudging with sage or using sound, such as bells or singing bowls, to cleanse and purify the energy. By clearing the energy field, one can create space for emotional healing and promote a sense of lightness and clarity.

3. EFT (Emotional Freedom Techniques): EFT, also known as tapping, combines elements of traditional Chinese medicine and psychotherapy. By tapping on specific acupressure points on the body, EFT aims to release emotional blockages and promote emotional well-being. This technique can be used to address a wide range of emotions, including anxiety, fear, and sadness.

4. Chakra Balancing: Chakras are energy centers within the body that are associated with different emotions and aspects of well-being. Balancing the chakras involves assessing and harmonizing the energy flow within each chakra. By addressing imbalances in the chakras, emotional healing and well-being can be facilitated.

5. Breathwork: Conscious breathing techniques can have a profound impact on emotional healing. Deep, intentional breathing can help release tension, promote relaxation, and create a sense of inner calm. Breathwork practices, such as Pranayama, can be incorporated into daily routines to support emotional well-being.

6. Meditation and Mindfulness: Meditation and mindfulness practices cultivate present-moment awareness and promote emotional balance. By focusing attention on the breath, sensations in the body, or the present moment, individuals can develop a greater sense of emotional resilience and reduce emotional reactivity.

The benefits of energy medicine in emotional healing are multifaceted. By addressing energetic imbalances, energy medicine techniques can support emotional release, reduce stress, and enhance emotional resilience. These techniques can also promote a greater sense of self-awareness and self-empowerment, allowing individuals to take an active role in their emotional well-being.

Moreover, energy medicine acknowledges the interplay between the physical, emotional, mental, and spiritual aspects of an individual. By working with the body's energy system, energy medicine provides a holistic framework for emotional healing, recognizing that true healing encompasses the integration of all these dimensions.

It is important to note that energy medicine techniques can complement but not replace traditional therapeutic approaches. They can be used alongside psychotherapy, counseling, or other forms of emotional support to enhance the healing process. Individuals seeking emotional healing should consult with qualified practitioners and professionals to ensure a holistic and integrated approach to their well-being.

Emotional Freedom Techniques (EFT)

Emotional Freedom Techniques (EFT), also known as tapping, is a powerful and innovative approach within the realm of energy medicine that aims to release emotional blockages and promote emotional well-being. Grounded in the principles of traditional Chinese medicine and modern psychology, EFT combines gentle tapping on specific acupressure points with focused attention on emotional issues. Below we will explore the principles, techniques, and benefits of EFT in relation to energy medicine.

EFT is based on the belief that emotional distress and imbalances can disrupt the body's energy system, leading to physical discomfort, mental distress, and emotional turmoil. By stimulating specific acupressure points while focusing on emotional issues, EFT aims to restore balance to the body's energy system and promote emotional healing.

The technique involves a sequence of tapping on various acupressure points located on the face, torso, and hands. These points are associated with the body's energy meridians, which are channels through which energy flows. By tapping on these points, it is believed that the flow of energy is restored, and emotional blockages are released.

During an EFT session, individuals identify and verbalize specific emotional issues or challenges they are facing. This could include fears, anxieties, past traumas, or negative beliefs. While stating the issue, the individual simultaneously taps on the acupressure points, following a specific sequence.

The tapping process is typically repeated several times while focusing on the emotional issue at hand. As individuals tap on the acupressure points, they may experience a release of emotions, sensations, or insights. The goal is to reduce the emotional intensity associated with the issue and promote a sense of emotional well-being.

EFT has been used to address a wide range of emotional concerns, including anxiety, stress, phobias, trauma, grief, and low self-esteem. It can also be applied to enhance performance in various areas of life, such as sports, public speaking, or creative endeavors. EFT is known for its ability to rapidly alleviate emotional distress and promote a greater sense of inner peace and resilience.

The benefits of EFT extend beyond the immediate relief of emotional distress. By working with the body's energy system, EFT can facilitate deeper emotional healing and promote long-term emotional well-being. It can help individuals release negative emotions, reframe limiting beliefs, and cultivate self-acceptance and self-compassion.

Moreover, EFT is a portable and self-empowering technique that individuals can use on their own to manage their emotional well-being. Once familiar with the technique, individuals can apply EFT as a self-help tool whenever they encounter emotional challenges or stressful situations. This accessibility makes EFT a valuable resource for emotional support and personal growth.

Research on EFT has shown promising results in various areas, including anxiety disorders, post-traumatic stress disorder (PTSD), phobias, and depression. Studies have demonstrated its effectiveness in reducing symptoms and improving emotional well-being. EFT has also been found to have a positive impact on physiological markers, such as heart rate variability and cortisol levels, indicating its influence on the body's stress response.

It is important to note that while EFT is generally safe and well-tolerated, it is not a substitute for professional mental health care. Individuals with complex or severe emotional issues should seek guidance from qualified professionals. EFT can be used as a complementary technique alongside traditional therapies to enhance the healing process.

The role of energy medicine in trauma release

Traumatic experiences can leave deep emotional and psychological imprints, affecting individuals long after the actual event has occurred. Energy medicine, with its holistic and integrative approach, offers valuable tools for trauma release and healing. By recognizing the interconnectedness of the mind, body, and energy system, energy medicine provides a unique perspective and a range of techniques to support individuals in their journey towards healing and recovery. Below we will explore the role of energy medicine in trauma release, highlighting its principles, techniques, and benefits.

Trauma is not solely an emotional or psychological phenomenon; it also impacts the body's energy system. When a traumatic event occurs, the body's natural energy flow can become disrupted or blocked, leading to physical, emotional, and energetic imbalances. Energy medicine approaches trauma from the perspective that by working with the body's energy system, these imbalances can be addressed, and healing can occur on multiple levels.

One of the key principles in energy medicine is the understanding that the body has an innate capacity to heal itself. By engaging with the body's energy system, energy medicine techniques aim to activate and support the body's self-healing mechanisms. These techniques focus on restoring balance, releasing blocked energy, and promoting the free flow of energy throughout the body.

Energy medicine offers a variety of techniques that can be effective in trauma release:

2. EFT (Emotional Freedom Techniques): EFT, also known as tapping, combines acupressure points with focused attention on emotional issues. By tapping on specific points while verbalizing the traumatic event or associated emotions, EFT aims to release emotional blockages and promote emotional well-being. This technique has been shown to be effective in reducing symptoms of trauma, anxiety, and stress.

3. Somatic Experiencing: Somatic Experiencing is a body-oriented approach to trauma healing developed by Peter A. Levine. It focuses on the physiological and sensory aspects of trauma, recognizing that trauma is stored in the body. Through gentle exercises and awareness of bodily sensations, Somatic Experiencing aims to discharge and regulate the energy that has become dysregulated during a traumatic event.

4. Breathwork: Conscious breathing techniques can be instrumental in trauma release. Deep, intentional breathing can help release tension, promote relaxation, and create a sense of safety within the body. By engaging with the breath, individuals can activate the body's relaxation response, facilitating the release of trauma-related energy and promoting emotional healing.

5. EMDR (Eye Movement Desensitization and Reprocessing): EMDR is a psychotherapy approach that incorporates elements of energy medicine. It involves bilateral stimulation of the brain through eye movements, sounds, or tactile sensations while recalling traumatic memories. This technique aims to reprocess and integrate traumatic experiences, facilitating healing and reducing distressing symptoms.

6. Energy Healing: Energy healing modalities, such as Reiki or Healing Touch, work with the body's energy field to promote balance, relaxation, and the release of blocked energy. These techniques can create a safe and supportive environment for individuals to process and release traumatic experiences, facilitating healing on multiple levels.

The benefits of energy medicine in trauma release are manifold. By addressing the energetic imbalances associated with trauma, individuals can experience a reduction in emotional distress, anxiety, and physical symptoms. Energy medicine techniques can help individuals regain a sense of safety, promote emotional regulation, and restore a positive sense of self.

Moreover, energy medicine recognizes that trauma is a complex and multidimensional experience. It acknowledges the impact of trauma on an individual's energetic and spiritual well-being. Energy medicine techniques can support individuals in reconnecting with their inner resources, fostering resilience, and promoting spiritual growth.

It is important to note that energy medicine approaches to trauma release should be used

Energy psychology and its applications

Energy psychology is a dynamic and evolving field within the realm of energy medicine that explores the relationship between the mind, body, and energy system. It encompasses a range of approaches that integrate psychological principles with techniques from traditional healing systems and modern energy medicine. Below we will explore the principles, techniques, and applications of energy psychology in relation to energy medicine.

Energy psychology operates on the understanding that the body's energy system plays a significant role in emotional and psychological well-being. It recognizes that disruptions or imbalances within the energy system can contribute to emotional distress and mental health issues. By addressing these energetic imbalances, energy psychology techniques aim to promote emotional healing and enhance psychological well-being.

One of the core principles of energy psychology is that the mind and body are interconnected, and changes in one affect the other. The techniques used in energy psychology often involve focused attention, intention, and specific actions that work with the body's energy system to influence the mind and emotions. By engaging with the energy system, individuals can access deeper levels of healing and transformation.

Energy psychology encompasses a variety of techniques and approaches, including:

2. Emotional Freedom Techniques (EFT): EFT, also known as tapping, combines elements of traditional Chinese medicine and modern psychology. By tapping on specific acupressure points while focusing on emotion-

al issues, EFT aims to release emotional blockages and promote emotional well-being. It has been used to address a wide range of emotional concerns, including anxiety, trauma, phobias, and stress.

3. Thought Field Therapy (TFT): TFT involves tapping on specific acupressure points in a specific sequence while focusing on a particular issue or belief. This technique aims to reprogram the body's energy system to eliminate negative emotions or beliefs. TFT has been used to address anxiety, trauma, addiction, and performance-related issues.

4. Psych-K: Psych-K is a technique that combines elements of psychology, neuroscience, and energy medicine. It involves a process of identifying and transforming subconscious beliefs that may be limiting or causing emotional distress. By using specific protocols and muscle testing, individuals can reprogram their subconscious mind to support positive beliefs and behaviors.

5. The Body Code: The Body Code is a comprehensive system that identifies and releases imbalances within the body's energy system. It utilizes muscle testing and a series of charts to identify energetic imbalances related to emotions, organs, systems, and other aspects of well-being. By releasing these imbalances, individuals can experience emotional healing and overall well-being.

The applications of energy psychology are broad and diverse. It can be used to address various psychological concerns, including anxiety disorders, phobias, post-traumatic stress disorder (PTSD), depression, and self-esteem issues. Energy psychology techniques are also effective in managing stress, improving performance, enhancing creativity, and promoting personal growth.

Energy psychology techniques can be utilized as standalone therapies or integrated with other therapeutic approaches, including counseling, psychotherapy, and energy medicine modalities. They can be used in individual sessions or in group settings, and they can be self-administered once individuals are familiar with the techniques.

The benefits of energy psychology extend beyond the immediate relief of symptoms. By addressing energetic imbalances and transforming negative beliefs or emotions, energy psychology techniques promote long-lasting changes in one's perception, behavior, and emotional well-being. They empower individuals to take an active role in their own healing and personal growth.

While energy psychology has gained recognition and popularity, it is important to note that research is still ongoing to validate its effectiveness and mechanisms of action. However, the growing body of evidence and the positive experiences reported by individuals and practitioners highlight the potential of energy psychology as a valuable tool in promoting psychological well-being.

Chapter Six

Energy Medicine and Chronic Illness

Chronic illnesses, such as autoimmune disorders, fibromyalgia, and chronic pain conditions, pose significant challenges to individuals' well-being and quality of life. Traditional medical approaches often focus on symptom management, but energy medicine offers a unique perspective and alternative strategies for addressing the underlying energetic imbalances associated with chronic illness. Below we will explore the principles, techniques, and benefits of energy medicine in relation to chronic illness.

At the heart of energy medicine is the understanding that the body is composed of a complex energy system that influences overall health and well-being. This energy system includes various aspects, such as the electromagnetic field, energy centers (chakras), and energy pathways (meridians). In the context of chronic illness, energy medicine recognizes that disruptions or imbalances within this energy system can contribute to the development and progression of disease.

Energy medicine approaches chronic illness from a holistic perspective, recognizing the interplay between physical, emotional, and energetic aspects of health. These approaches aim to restore balance, enhance vitality, and activate the body's self-healing mechanisms. By addressing energetic imbalances, energy medicine offers a comprehensive and integrative approach to chronic illness management.

Several energy medicine techniques can be applied in the context of chronic illness:

2. Rebalancing the Energy System: Energy medicine techniques, such as acupuncture, acupressure, or hands-on energy healing modalities, aim to rebalance the body's energy system. These techniques promote the free flow of energy throughout the body, addressing energy blockages and restoring energetic harmony. By enhancing the flow of energy, the body's innate healing mechanisms can be activated, supporting overall well-being.

3. Chakra Balancing: Chakras are energy centers within the body that are associated with different aspects of health and well-being. Chronic illness can be related to imbalances in specific chakras. Through techniques such as meditation, visualization, or energy healing, individuals can restore balance to the chakra system, supporting the body's natural healing processes.

4. Mind-Body Techniques: Chronic illness often involves a complex interplay between physical symptoms and emotional or psychological factors. Mind-body techniques, such as meditation, guided imagery, or breathwork, can be integrated into a comprehensive treatment plan. These techniques promote relaxation, stress reduction, and emotional well-being, positively influencing the body's response to chronic illness.

5. Energetic Clearing: Chronic illness can be associated with stagnant or dense energy in the body. Energetic clearing techniques, such as smudging, sound healing, or energy cleansing practices, aim to release and clear this stagnant energy. By creating a harmonious energetic environment, these practices support the body's natural healing processes.

The benefits of energy medicine in chronic illness management are multifaceted. By addressing energetic imbalances, these approaches can complement traditional medical treatments, promoting overall well-being and potentially enhancing the effectiveness of other therapies. Energy medicine techniques have been reported to reduce pain, alleviate symptoms, improve energy levels, and enhance quality of life in individuals with chronic illnesses.

Moreover, energy medicine provides individuals with chronic illnesses a sense of empowerment and active participation in their healing journey. By engaging with their energy system, individuals can cultivate self-awareness, develop self-care practices, and take an active role in their well-being. This shift towards self-empowerment can positively impact their emotional and psychological outlook, contributing to improved coping skills and resilience.

It is important to note that energy medicine approaches should not be seen as a replacement for conventional medical care. They should be used as complementary strategies to enhance overall well-being and support the body's self-healing capacities. It is essential to consult with qualified practitioners and healthcare professionals to ensure a comprehensive and integrative approach to chronic illness management.

Managing pain with energy medicine

1. Managing Pain with Energy Medicine: Harnessing the Power of Energy for Relief

Pain is a complex and multi-faceted experience that affects millions of people worldwide. While conventional approaches to pain management typically involve medication and physical therapies, energy medicine offers an alternative perspective and a range of techniques for addressing pain at its energetic source. Below we will explore the principles, techniques, and benefits of energy medicine in relation to pain management.

At the core of energy medicine is the recognition that pain is not only a physical sensation but also an energetic manifestation. It acknowledges that imbalances or blockages in the body's energy system can contribute to the experience of pain. By addressing these energetic imbalances, energy medicine techniques aim to alleviate pain and support overall well-being.

Energy medicine approaches pain management from a holistic perspective, recognizing the interconnectedness of the physical, emotional, and energetic aspects of pain. These approaches focus on restoring balance, promoting the free flow of energy, and activating the body's self-healing mechanisms. By working with the body's energy system, energy medicine offers a comprehensive and integrative approach to pain management.

Several energy medicine techniques can be effective in managing pain:

2. Acupuncture and Acupressure: Acupuncture and acupressure are based on the principles of traditional Chinese medicine, which recognize the existence of energy meridians and acupoints in the body. By stimulating specific acupoints, these techniques aim to regulate the flow of energy and promote pain relief. Acupuncture involves the insertion of fine needles into acupoints, while acupressure applies pressure to these points using fingers or other devices.

3. Reiki and Healing Touch: Reiki and Healing Touch are energy healing modalities that involve the gentle placement of hands on or near the body. These techniques aim to balance and harmonize the body's energy, promoting relaxation, reducing stress, and relieving pain. The practitioner serves as a conduit for healing energy, facilitating the flow of energy to areas of pain or discomfort.

4. Pulsed Electromagnetic Field Therapy (PEMF): PEMF involves the application of specific frequencies and intensities of electromagnetic fields to the body. These fields can penetrate deep into the tissues, stimulating

cellular repair and reducing inflammation. PEMF has shown promising results in managing pain associated with various conditions, including arthritis, fibromyalgia, and sports injuries.

5. Mind-Body Techniques: Mind-body techniques, such as meditation, mindfulness, and breathwork, can be powerful tools in pain management. These techniques promote relaxation, reduce stress, and enhance self-awareness, allowing individuals to cultivate a sense of inner calm and develop a positive relationship with pain. By shifting their perception and response to pain, individuals can experience relief and improved well-being.

6. EFT (Emotional Freedom Techniques): EFT combines acupressure with focused attention on emotional issues or physical sensations. By tapping on specific acupoints while verbalizing pain-related statements, EFT aims to release emotional blockages and promote pain relief. This technique has been found to be effective in managing various types of pain, including chronic pain and pain associated with emotional trauma.

The benefits of energy medicine in pain management are significant. By addressing energetic imbalances and promoting the free flow of energy, these approaches can complement conventional pain management strategies, potentially reducing the need for high doses of medication and their associated side effects. Energy medicine techniques have been reported to reduce pain intensity, improve pain tolerance, enhance overall well-being, and promote a greater sense of self-control and empowerment.

Furthermore, energy medicine provides individuals with pain a sense of active participation in their healing process. By engaging with their energy system, individuals can develop self-care practices, learn to listen to their body's needs, and take an active role in managing their pain

The role of energy medicine in cancer treatment

1. The Role of Energy Medicine in Cancer Treatment: Exploring Complementary Approaches to Healing

Cancer, one of the most prevalent diseases of our time, requires a multidimensional approach to treatment and healing. While conventional cancer treatments like chemotherapy, radiation, and surgery are essential, there is a growing recognition of the potential benefits of complementary approaches, including energy medicine. Energy medicine offers a unique perspective and a range of techniques that can support individuals undergoing cancer treatment. Below we will explore the principles, techniques, and potential benefits of energy medicine in relation to cancer treatment.

Energy medicine views the body as a dynamic energy system, with the understanding that imbalances or disruptions in this energy system can contribute to the development and progression of disease. Cancer, in particular, is seen as a complex interplay of physical, emotional, and energetic factors. Energy medicine approaches cancer treatment from a holistic perspective, aiming to restore balance, promote vitality, and activate the body's self-healing mechanisms.

One of the key principles of energy medicine is the recognition that energy flows through the body along specific pathways or meridians. These meridians are believed to carry vital life force energy, and any blockages or imbalances can affect the overall well-being of an individual. By working with the body's energy system, energy medicine techniques aim to restore the free flow of energy, enhancing the body's ability to heal and recover.

Several energy medicine techniques can be beneficial in cancer treatment:

2. Acupuncture and Acupressure: Acupuncture and acupressure are ancient practices rooted in traditional Chinese medicine. By stimulating

specific acupoints along the body's meridians, these techniques aim to restore balance, promote energy flow, and support overall well-being. In cancer treatment, acupuncture and acupressure have been used to alleviate treatment-related side effects such as pain, nausea, fatigue, and anxiety.

3. Reiki and Healing Touch: Reiki and Healing Touch are energy healing modalities that involve the gentle placement of hands on or near the body. These techniques aim to balance and harmonize the body's energy, promoting relaxation, reducing stress, and supporting the body's healing processes. In cancer treatment, Reiki and Healing Touch have been used to enhance overall well-being, reduce treatment-related side effects, and provide emotional support.

4. Visualization and Guided Imagery: Visualization and guided imagery are techniques that utilize the power of the mind to create positive healing experiences. These techniques involve creating vivid mental images of healing and recovery, promoting relaxation and positive emotional states. In cancer treatment, visualization and guided imagery have been used to reduce anxiety, manage pain, and enhance the effectiveness of conventional treatments.

5. Mind-Body Techniques: Mind-body techniques, such as meditation, mindfulness, and breathwork, can be valuable tools in cancer treatment. These techniques promote relaxation, reduce stress, and enhance self-awareness, supporting individuals in coping with the challenges of cancer treatment. Mind-body approaches have been shown to improve quality of life, reduce anxiety and depression, and enhance immune function in cancer patients.

6. EFT (Emotional Freedom Techniques): EFT combines acupressure with focused attention on emotional issues. By tapping on specific acupoints while addressing emotional challenges or physical symptoms, EFT

aims to release emotional blockages and promote overall well-being. In cancer treatment, EFT has been used to alleviate emotional distress, reduce treatment-related side effects, and support emotional healing.

The benefits of energy medicine in cancer treatment are diverse. These techniques can complement conventional treatments, providing individuals with a sense of control and empowerment, and potentially reducing treatment-related side effects. Energy medicine techniques have been reported to improve overall well-being, reduce pain and discomfort, enhance emotional resilience, and promote a positive outlook.

It is essential to note that

Energy medicine for autoimmune disorders

1. Energy Medicine for Autoimmune Disorders: Nurturing Balance and Harmony within the Body

Autoimmune disorders are complex conditions in which the immune system mistakenly attacks healthy cells and tissues. These disorders can have a profound impact on an individual's quality of life and often require long-term management. While conventional medicine focuses on symptom management and immune suppression, energy medicine offers a holistic and integrative approach to support individuals with autoimmune disorders. Below we will explore the principles, techniques, and potential benefits of energy medicine in relation to autoimmune disorders.

Energy medicine recognizes that the body is not only composed of physical matter but also of subtle energy fields that influence overall health and well-being. It views autoimmune disorders as disruptions or imbalances within the body's energy system. By addressing these energetic imbalances, energy medicine techniques aim to restore balance, promote vitality, and activate the body's self-healing mechanisms.

One of the central principles of energy medicine is that the body has an innate ability to heal itself. By engaging with the body's energy system, energy medicine techniques seek to activate and support the body's self-regulation and self-repair mechanisms. These techniques focus on balancing the body's energy, addressing energy blockages, and enhancing the overall flow of energy.

Several energy medicine techniques can be beneficial in managing autoimmune disorders:

2. Acupuncture and Acupressure: Acupuncture and acupressure are traditional Chinese medicine practices that work with the body's energy meridians and acupoints. By stimulating specific points along these meridians, these techniques aim to restore the flow of energy, strengthen the immune system, and promote overall well-being. Acupuncture and acupressure have been used in the management of various autoimmune disorders, including rheumatoid arthritis, lupus, and multiple sclerosis.

3. Reiki and Healing Touch: Reiki and Healing Touch are energy healing modalities that involve the gentle placement of hands on or near the body. These techniques aim to balance and harmonize the body's energy, promote relaxation, reduce stress, and support the body's healing processes. In the context of autoimmune disorders, Reiki and Healing Touch have been used to support overall well-being, alleviate pain and inflammation, and provide emotional support.

4. Mind-Body Techniques: Mind-body techniques, such as meditation, mindfulness, and breathwork, can be valuable tools in managing autoimmune disorders. These techniques promote relaxation, reduce stress, and enhance self-awareness, supporting individuals in coping with the physi-

cal and emotional challenges associated with these disorders. Mind-body approaches have been shown to reduce inflammation, improve immune function, and enhance overall well-being in individuals with autoimmune conditions.

5. Dietary and Nutritional Support: Energy medicine approaches to autoimmune disorders often emphasize the importance of diet and nutrition. Certain foods and dietary factors can contribute to inflammation and immune dysregulation. Energy medicine practitioners may offer guidance on adopting an anti-inflammatory diet, incorporating specific nutrients, and identifying food sensitivities or intolerances that may exacerbate autoimmune symptoms.

6. Energetic Clearing: Energetic clearing techniques aim to release stagnant or negative energy from the body's energy field. These techniques may include practices such as smudging, sound healing, or energy cleansing rituals. By clearing the energy field, these practices create a more harmonious energetic environment and support the body's natural healing processes.

The benefits of energy medicine in managing autoimmune disorders are multifaceted. By addressing energetic imbalances and promoting the free flow of energy, energy medicine techniques can complement conventional medical treatments, potentially reducing the need for high doses of medication and their associated side effects. Energy medicine approaches have been reported to reduce pain and inflammation, improve immune function, enhance overall well-being, and support emotional resilience.

It is important to note that energy medicine approaches should not be seen as a replacement for

Supporting mental health with energy medicine

1. Supporting Mental Health with Energy Medicine: Nurturing Emotional Well-Being

Mental health is a vital aspect of overall well-being, and maintaining emotional balance is essential for leading a fulfilling life. While conventional approaches to mental health often focus on medication and psychotherapy, energy medicine offers alternative perspectives and techniques for supporting mental and emotional well-being. Below we will explore the principles, techniques, and potential benefits of energy medicine in relation to mental health.

Energy medicine recognizes the intimate connection between the mind, body, and energy system. It views mental health issues as manifestations of imbalances or disruptions within the body's energy system. By addressing these energetic imbalances, energy medicine techniques aim to restore harmony, promote emotional well-being, and activate the body's self-healing mechanisms.

One of the core principles of energy medicine is that the body has an innate ability to heal itself. By engaging with the body's energy system, energy medicine techniques seek to activate and support the body's self-regulation and self-repair mechanisms. These techniques focus on balancing the body's energy, releasing blockages, and promoting the free flow of energy.

Several energy medicine techniques can be beneficial in supporting mental health:

2. EFT (Emotional Freedom Techniques): EFT, also known as tapping, combines acupressure with focused attention on emotional issues. By tapping on specific acupoints while addressing emotional challenges or negative beliefs, EFT aims to release emotional blockages, reduce stress, and promote emotional well-being. It has been used to address a wide range

of mental health concerns, including anxiety, depression, post-traumatic stress disorder (PTSD), and phobias.

3. Reiki and Healing Touch: Reiki and Healing Touch are energy healing modalities that involve the gentle placement of hands on or near the body. These techniques aim to balance and harmonize the body's energy, promote relaxation, reduce stress, and support emotional well-being. In the context of mental health, Reiki and Healing Touch have been used to alleviate anxiety, depression, and emotional distress, providing individuals with a sense of calm and promoting overall well-being.

4. Chakra Balancing: Chakras are energy centers within the body that are associated with different emotions and aspects of well-being. Balancing the chakras involves assessing and harmonizing the flow of energy within each chakra. By addressing imbalances in the chakras, energy medicine techniques can support emotional healing and promote overall mental well-being.

5. Mind-Body Techniques: Mind-body techniques, such as meditation, mindfulness, and breathwork, play a significant role in supporting mental health. These techniques promote relaxation, reduce stress, and enhance self-awareness, allowing individuals to cultivate a sense of inner calm and emotional resilience. Mind-body approaches have been shown to reduce symptoms of anxiety, depression, and other mental health conditions, improving overall well-being and quality of life.

6. Energetic Clearing: Energetic clearing techniques aim to release stagnant or negative energy from the body's energy field. These techniques may include practices such as smudging, sound healing, or energy cleansing rituals. By clearing the energy field, these practices create a more harmonious energetic environment, supporting emotional well-being and promoting a sense of clarity and balance.

The benefits of energy medicine in supporting mental health are diverse. By addressing energetic imbalances and promoting the free flow of energy, energy medicine techniques can complement conventional mental health treatments, potentially reducing the need for high doses of medication and their associated side effects. Energy medicine approaches have been reported to reduce symptoms of anxiety, depression, and emotional distress, improve emotional resilience, and support personal growth and self-empowerment.

It is important to note that energy medicine approaches should not be seen as a replacement for conventional mental health care

Chapter Seven

The Science of Energy Medicine

Energy medicine is a fascinating and rapidly evolving field that explores the role of subtle energy in promoting health and well-being. While the concept of energy healing may seem mystical or esoteric, there is a growing body of scientific research that supports the efficacy of energy medicine modalities. Below we will delve into the science behind energy medicine, examining the principles, research findings, and potential mechanisms of action that underlie this intriguing field.

At the heart of energy medicine is the recognition that the human body is composed of a complex energy system. This system includes the flow of bioelectricity, electromagnetic fields, and subtle energies that interact with the physical body. Energy medicine approaches aim to harness and balance these energies to facilitate healing and promote overall well-being.

One area of scientific research that contributes to our understanding of energy medicine is the study of bioelectricity. The body generates and conducts electrical impulses through the nervous system, muscular contractions, and the movement of ions across cell membranes. This bioelectricity plays a crucial role in cellular communication, tissue regeneration, and immune function. Techniques such as acupuncture and acupressure are believed to modulate this bioelectricity, promoting the flow of energy along specific pathways and facilitating healing.

Another area of research relevant to energy medicine is the study of electromagnetic fields. The body generates and is influenced by various electromagnetic fields, including the heart's electromagnetic field and the brain's electrical activity. These fields can interact with external electromagnetic fields, such as those emitted by electronic devices or the Earth's magnetic field. Research suggests that electromagnetic fields can affect cellular processes, regulate gene expression, and influence physiological functions. Energy medicine techniques like PEMF (Pulsed Electromagnetic Field Therapy) utilize these principles to promote healing and alleviate pain.

One intriguing aspect of energy medicine is the phenomenon of the human energy field. Research using technologies like Kirlian photography, gas discharge visualization, and biofield imaging has provided visual evidence of the energy field surrounding the body. This field is believed to contain information about an individual's physical, emotional, and energetic state. Energy medicine modalities such as Reiki and Healing Touch aim to balance and manipulate this field to facilitate healing and promote overall well-being.

Quantum physics also provides a framework for understanding energy medicine. The principles of quantum physics suggest that at the fundamental level, everything is composed of energy and is interconnected. Quantum entanglement, for example, describes how particles can become linked regardless of distance, implying a non-local and instantaneous communication. Energy medicine acknowledges the interconnectedness of all aspects of existence and aims to work with this inherent unity to restore balance and harmony.

While the scientific understanding of energy medicine is still evolving, research has yielded promising findings. Studies have demonstrated the effectiveness of energy medicine modalities in various areas, including pain management, wound healing, stress reduction, and immune system enhancement. For example, randomized controlled trials have shown the positive effects of acupuncture on pain relief, and studies using biofield therapies have demonstrated improved wound healing rates. Furthermore, research has revealed physiological changes associated with energy medicine, such as altered brainwave patterns and changes in heart rate variability.

The mechanisms through which energy medicine works are still being explored. One proposed mechanism is the modulation of the body's bioelectric and electromagnetic fields, influencing cellular processes and promoting self-regulation. Additionally, energy medicine modalities may stimulate the release of endorphins and other neurotransmitters, promoting pain relief and emotional well-being. The relaxation response induced by energy medicine techniques can also have profound effects on the nervous system, immune system, and stress hormone levels.

It is important to note that energy medicine is not meant to replace conventional medical care but to complement it. Energy medicine approaches can work in synergy with traditional therapies, supporting the

Quantum physics and energy medicine

Quantum physics, the branch of science that studies the behavior of matter and energy at the smallest scales, has revolutionized our understanding of the universe. It has also shed light on the underlying principles of energy medicine, a field that explores the role of subtle energy in healing and well-being. Below we will delve into the fascinating relationship between quantum physics and energy medicine, exploring how the principles of quantum physics relate to the concepts and practices of energy medicine.

One of the fundamental principles of quantum physics is the recognition that everything in the universe, including matter and energy, is composed of particles and waves. These particles, such as electrons and photons, exhibit both particle-like and wave-like behavior, challenging the traditional notion of separate, solid entities. Instead, particles are considered to exist in a state of superposition, where they can simultaneously occupy multiple positions or states until observed or measured.

This principle of superposition is relevant to energy medicine as it suggests that reality is not fixed but rather a fluid and dynamic field of possibilities. Energy medicine recognizes that health and well-being are not solely determined by the physical body but are influenced by the subtle energy systems and the interconnectedness of mind, body, and spirit. By working with the body's energy systems, energy medicine techniques aim to influence the flow and interaction of these subtle energies to promote healing and balance.

Another key principle of quantum physics is the phenomenon of entanglement, which describes how particles become connected or correlated regardless of distance. When particles are entangled, the state of one particle instantaneously affects the state of the other, even if they are separated by vast distances. This concept challenges the traditional understanding of cause and effect and implies a non-local, interconnected nature of reality.

Energy medicine embraces the idea of interconnectedness and non-locality. It recognizes that subtle energy fields extend beyond the physical body and interact with the environment and other living beings. Energy medicine modalities like Reiki, Healing Touch, and distant healing techniques are based on the belief that intentions, thoughts, and energetic interventions can have an effect on the well-being of individuals, regardless of physical proximity.

The concept of the observer effect in quantum physics is also relevant to energy medicine. According to the observer effect, the act of observing or measuring a quantum system can affect its behavior. This suggests that consciousness plays a role in shaping reality. Energy medicine approaches acknowledge the influence of consciousness and intention in healing. Practitioners and individuals engage in focused intention, visualization, and directing energy with the intention of promoting healing and balance within the body's energy systems.

Quantum physics also highlights the importance of the underlying energy and information fields that exist beyond the physical realm. The concept of the zero-point field, for instance, suggests that even in a vacuum, space is not empty but filled with energy fluctuations. This energy field contains vast amounts of information and potential. Energy medicine modalities tap into this field, accessing and channeling the subtle energies to support healing and promote well-being.

It is important to note that while the principles of quantum physics offer intriguing insights into the nature of reality, the application of these principles to energy medicine is an ongoing area of exploration and debate. The field of quantum biology, for instance, investigates how quantum processes may operate within living organisms. Research is also being conducted to understand the mechanisms through which energy medicine modalities influence the body's energy systems and promote healing.

The placebo effect and the power of belief

The placebo effect is a phenomenon that has long fascinated scientists and researchers. It refers to the remarkable ability of the human mind to elicit healing responses when presented with inert substances or sham treatments. While traditionally viewed as a deceptive response, the placebo effect now stands as a testament to the power of belief and the mind's influence on the body's healing mechanisms. In the realm of energy medicine, understanding the placebo effect is crucial, as it highlights the role of belief and intention in promoting healing and well-being. Below we will explore the placebo effect and its relationship to energy medicine.

The placebo effect operates on the principle that the mind and body are interconnected, constantly communicating and influencing one another. When a person believes they are receiving a treatment or intervention, the mind engages the body's healing resources, often resulting in noticeable improvements in symptoms or overall well-being. The placebo effect is not limited to the realm of pharmaceuticals; it can also be observed in various interventions, including energy medicine techniques.

Energy medicine modalities harness the power of belief and intention, recognizing that these factors play a vital role in promoting healing. Techniques such as Reiki, Healing Touch, and acupuncture utilize the principles of energy flow and intention to facilitate balance and well-being. When individuals believe in the efficacy of these interventions and have positive expectations, their belief systems interact with the body's energy systems, potentially leading to significant healing responses.

Research has demonstrated the influence of belief on the placebo effect. Studies have shown that individuals who receive a placebo treatment, while believing it to be a genuine intervention, often experience reductions in pain, improvements in symptoms, and overall better outcomes compared to those who receive no treatment. This highlights the significant impact of belief and positive expectations on the body's healing responses.

The mechanisms underlying the placebo effect are multifaceted and not yet fully understood. One proposed explanation is that belief and expectation activate certain regions of the brain, triggering the release of endorphins and other neurotransmitters associated with pain relief and well-being. These neurochemical changes can lead to physiological changes and improved health outcomes.

Furthermore, belief and expectation can influence the body's stress response. When individuals have positive beliefs and expectations about a treatment or intervention, it can reduce stress and anxiety levels, allowing the body to shift into a state of relaxation and healing. This, in turn, can positively impact various physiological processes, such as immune function and inflammation regulation.

The placebo effect also highlights the importance of the therapeutic relationship and the context in which healing interventions are administered. Factors such as a compassionate and supportive practitioner, a nurturing environment, and positive communication can enhance the placebo effect. In energy medicine, practitioners often cultivate a healing space that promotes trust, relaxation, and positive expectations, further amplifying the potential healing responses.

The placebo effect serves as a reminder of the intricate mind-body connection and the capacity for self-healing. It challenges the notion that healing solely depends on external interventions and emphasizes the role of the individual's beliefs and internal resources. The mind's influence on the body's healing responses can be harnessed and optimized through techniques that cultivate positive beliefs, intentions, and expectations.

However, it is important to note that the placebo effect should not be seen as a replacement for evidence-based medical interventions. The placebo effect is most effective in subjective experiences, such as pain relief, symptom improvement, and well-being enhancement. It does not eradicate the need for rigorous scientific research and appropriate medical care. Nonetheless, it highlights the potential of belief and intention as powerful allies in the healing process.

Measuring and validating energy medicine practices

Energy medicine, a field that explores the role of subtle energies in promoting health and well-being, has gained significant attention in recent years. While energy medicine techniques have been used for centuries, the scientific validation of these practices has been a subject of interest and inquiry. Measuring and validating energy medicine practices is crucial for establishing their credibility and expanding their integration into mainstream healthcare. Below we will explore the challenges and advancements in measuring and validating energy medicine practices.

One of the challenges in measuring energy medicine practices is the nature of subtle energies themselves. These energies are often described as biofields, electromagnetic fields, or vibrational frequencies. Unlike the measurable physical forces, such as gravity or magnetism, subtle energies are not easily detectable using conventional scientific instruments. Their effects may be subtle and difficult to quantify using traditional research methodologies.

Despite these challenges, there have been notable advancements in measuring and validating energy medicine practices. Researchers have utilized various tools and techniques to study the effects of energy medicine modalities. Some of the approaches include:

2. Biofield Imaging: Biofield imaging techniques, such as gas discharge visualization (GDV) and electro-photonic imaging (EPI), offer visual representations of the human energy field. These technologies capture and analyze the light emissions from the body, providing insights into the energy dynamics and interactions within the biofield. Biofield imaging has been used to investigate the effects of energy healing techniques and assess changes in the energy field before and after energy medicine interventions.

3. Physiological Measurements: Researchers have explored the physiological changes associated with energy medicine practices. Techniques such

as electroencephalography (EEG), heart rate variability (HRV), and skin conductance have been employed to assess changes in brainwave patterns, heart rate coherence, and autonomic nervous system activity. These measurements provide objective data on the physiological effects of energy medicine techniques.

4. Biomarkers and Biochemical Analysis: Energy medicine practices have been examined for their impact on specific biomarkers and biochemical parameters. Studies have investigated changes in immune markers, stress hormones, cytokine levels, and other biological indicators associated with healing and well-being. These measurements contribute to the scientific understanding of the mechanisms underlying energy medicine practices.

5. Randomized Controlled Trials (RCTs): RCTs are considered the gold standard for scientific research. They involve randomly assigning participants to treatment and control groups to evaluate the efficacy of interventions. Several RCTs have been conducted to assess the effects of energy medicine techniques, such as acupuncture, Reiki, and Healing Touch, on various health outcomes. These studies provide valuable evidence for the effectiveness of energy medicine practices.

In addition to measuring the physiological and biochemical effects, researchers have explored the psychosocial aspects of energy medicine practices. Qualitative research methods, including interviews and surveys, have been utilized to explore the experiences and subjective outcomes of individuals who have undergone energy medicine interventions. These qualitative insights shed light on the personal experiences and perceptions of those engaging in energy medicine practices.

Validation of energy medicine practices goes beyond measuring their immediate effects. Long-term studies assessing the sustained benefits and potential impact on disease progression are also essential. Longitudinal studies, cohort studies, and systematic reviews/meta-analyses are valuable research methodologies for evaluating the long-term effects of energy medicine practices and assessing their clinical significance.

While significant progress has been made in measuring and validating energy medicine practices, it is important to acknowledge the complexities and limitations of scientific research in this field. The subtle nature of energy, the diversity of energy medicine techniques, and the individualized responses to these practices pose challenges in designing and conducting rigorous studies. Additionally, the interdisciplinary nature of energy medicine requires collaboration between various scientific disciplines, including physics, biology, psychology, and medicine.

It is

Chapter Eight

Balancing Your Energy

Energy is the essence of life. It flows within us and around us, influencing our physical, mental, and emotional well-being. When our energy is in balance, we experience a sense of vitality, clarity, and harmony. However, daily stress, emotional challenges, and environmental factors can disrupt this delicate balance. Energy medicine offers a holistic approach to restoring and maintaining equilibrium within our energy system. Below we will explore the concept of balancing energy, the principles of energy medicine, and practical techniques for nurturing harmony and well-being.

Energy medicine recognizes that the human body is not merely a physical entity but also an intricate network of energy pathways and fields. These energy pathways, known as meridians or channels, facilitate the flow of life force energy, also referred to as chi, prana, or vital energy. When the flow of energy is smooth and unimpeded, we experience a state of balance and optimal functioning.

Imbalances in our energy system can manifest as physical, emotional, or mental symptoms. For example, blockages or disturbances in energy flow may contribute to feelings of fatigue, pain, anxiety, or irritability. Energy medicine techniques aim to address these imbalances and restore the harmonious flow of energy, supporting overall well-being.

One fundamental principle of energy medicine is that everything is energy, and energy is influenced by intention and attention. Our thoughts, emotions, and beliefs can have a profound impact on our energy system.

Negative thoughts, stress, and unresolved emotions can create energetic blockages, while positive thoughts and intentions can promote the free flow of energy.

Practitioners of energy medicine utilize various techniques to balance and harmonize the body's energy:

2. Acupuncture and Acupressure: These techniques, rooted in traditional Chinese medicine, involve stimulating specific points along the body's meridians to regulate energy flow. Acupuncture utilizes fine needles, while acupressure applies pressure with fingers or tools. Both approaches help release blockages, restore balance, and promote well-being.

3. Reiki and Healing Touch: These energy healing modalities involve the gentle placement of hands on or near the body. Practitioners act as conduits for healing energy, directing it to areas of imbalance or distress. Reiki and Healing Touch promote deep relaxation, stress reduction, and the restoration of energy flow.

4. Breathwork and Meditation: Conscious breathing techniques and meditation practices have been used for centuries to calm the mind, relax the body, and enhance the flow of energy. Deep, diaphragmatic breathing and mindfulness meditation support the release of tension, increase oxygenation, and foster a sense of inner calm and balance.

5. Movement Practices: Certain movement-based practices, such as qigong and tai chi, combine gentle physical movements with breath awareness to cultivate and balance energy. These practices promote relaxation, flexibility, and the flow of vital energy throughout the body.

6. Emotional Release Techniques: Emotional well-being is closely tied to energy balance. Emotional Freedom Techniques (EFT) and other similar approaches help release emotional blockages by tapping on specific acu-

points while addressing unresolved emotions or negative beliefs. These techniques promote emotional healing and support the flow of energy.

In addition to these specific techniques, cultivating a lifestyle that nurtures balance and well-being is essential for maintaining harmonious energy. Practices such as spending time in nature, engaging in creative activities, practicing gratitude, maintaining healthy relationships, and engaging in self-care routines contribute to overall energetic balance.

It is important to note that balancing energy is a dynamic process that requires self-awareness and regular practice. Each person's energy system is unique, and what works for one individual may not work for another. It is crucial to listen to your body's signals and choose techniques

Techniques for grounding and centering

In our fast-paced and chaotic world, it's easy to feel overwhelmed, scattered, and disconnected from our inner selves. Grounding and centering techniques offer a powerful remedy, helping us reconnect with our essence, find stability, and restore balance. These techniques, rooted in energy medicine, provide practical tools to navigate life's challenges with greater resilience and clarity. Below we will explore the concept of grounding and centering, the principles behind these techniques, and practical ways to incorporate them into our daily lives.

Grounding, also known as earthing, is the process of connecting our energy with the Earth's energy. It allows us to release excess energy and find stability, like the roots of a tree anchoring it to the ground. Centering, on the other hand, involves directing our focus and awareness inward, bringing our attention to the present moment and finding a sense of inner balance and calm.

Energy medicine acknowledges the significance of grounding and centering in maintaining overall well-being. When we are ungrounded or uncentered, we may experience feelings of anxiety, scattered thoughts, and difficulty in making decisions. Grounding and centering techniques help us feel rooted, connected, and in tune with our inner guidance.

Several techniques can assist in grounding and centering:

2. Grounding Visualization: Sit or stand with your feet firmly on the ground. Close your eyes and imagine roots growing from the soles of your feet, extending deep into the Earth. Visualize these roots absorbing nourishing energy from the Earth, and feel yourself becoming grounded and supported.

3. Barefoot Walking: Take off your shoes and spend some time walking barefoot on natural surfaces such as grass, sand, or soil. Pay attention to the sensations in your feet as they make contact with the Earth. This practice allows for a direct energetic connection between your body and the Earth's energy.

4. Breathwork: Focus on your breath as a means of grounding and centering. Take slow, deep breaths, inhaling through your nose and exhaling through your mouth. As you breathe, imagine inhaling a sense of stability and exhaling any tension or stress. This conscious breathing practice brings your attention to the present moment and helps calm the mind.

5. Body Scan Meditation: Lie down or sit in a comfortable position. Close your eyes and bring your awareness to different parts of your body, starting from your toes and gradually moving up to the top of your head. As you scan each area, release any tension or discomfort, allowing your body to relax and become grounded in the present moment.

6. Nature Connection: Spend time in nature to ground and center yourself. Whether it's sitting under a tree, walking in a park, or hiking in the mountains, immersing yourself in nature allows you to connect with the Earth's energy and find a sense of peace and balance.

7. Physical Movement: Engage in activities that promote body awareness and grounding, such as yoga, tai chi, or dance. These practices combine mindful movement, breath awareness, and grounding principles, helping to release stagnant energy and restore balance.

8. Sensory Awareness: Bring your attention to your senses to anchor yourself in the present moment. Notice the physical sensations, smells, sounds, and colors around you. Engaging your senses brings you into the here and now, promoting a sense of centeredness and presence.

9. Use of Crystals or Stones: Some people find that holding or carrying grounding crystals or stones, such as hematite, obsidian, or jasper, can enhance their grounding experience. These natural objects are believed to have stabilizing and grounding properties that resonate with our energy field.

By incorporating these techniques into our daily lives, we can enhance

Energy cleansing and protection

In our daily lives, we encounter various energies that can impact our well-being and vitality. Just as we cleanse our physical bodies to maintain hygiene and health, it is equally important to cleanse and protect our energy field. Energy cleansing and protection practices, rooted in energy medicine, offer effective tools to clear stagnant or negative energies and create a harmonious energetic environment. Below we will explore the concept of energy cleansing and protection, the principles behind these practices, and practical techniques to incorporate them into our lives.

Energy medicine recognizes that our energy field, also known as the aura or biofield, extends beyond the physical body and interacts with the environment. This field can accumulate energetic imprints from emotions, thoughts, interactions, and environmental factors. If left unattended, these imprints can create energetic blockages, leading to a sense of heaviness, fatigue, and emotional imbalance. Energy cleansing practices aim to clear these imprints and restore the natural flow of energy.

Additionally, energy protection practices shield our energy field from external influences and prevent energetic depletion. Just as we protect our physical bodies from harm, energy protection techniques safeguard our energy field, enabling us to navigate challenging situations with resilience and maintaining our energetic integrity.

Several techniques can assist in energy cleansing and protection:

2. Smudging: Smudging involves burning herbs, such as sage, cedar, or palo santo, and allowing the smoke to permeate the energy field. As the smoke wafts around, it is believed to purify the energy field by clearing negative or stagnant energies. Smudging is often performed in a ritualistic manner, accompanied by intentions and prayers.

3. Salt Baths or Showers: Salt is known for its purifying properties. Taking a bath or shower with sea salt or Epsom salt can cleanse the energy field and help release energetic debris. As you soak or shower, visualize the saltwater washing away any unwanted energies, leaving you feeling refreshed and rejuvenated.

4. Sound Healing: Sound has a profound impact on our energy field. Various instruments, such as singing bowls, tuning forks, or drums, can

be used to create harmonious vibrations that resonate with our energy field. The sounds produced during sound healing sessions are believed to dislodge stagnant energy and promote a sense of balance and well-being.

5. Energetic Clearing Rituals: Energetic clearing rituals involve consciously releasing negative or stagnant energy from the energy field. These rituals can include practices such as visualization, intention setting, and energy sweeping. During these rituals, individuals imagine a flow of cleansing energy passing through their energy field, sweeping away any unwanted energies and leaving behind a sense of lightness and clarity.

6. Crystal Cleansing: Crystals have unique energetic properties and can assist in energy cleansing. Placing crystals, such as clear quartz or selenite, in sunlight or moonlight can help clear their energetic imprints. Additionally, some people find that placing crystals on or near the body can absorb and transmute negative energies, promoting a sense of balance and protection.

7. Intention Setting: Intention is a powerful tool in energy medicine. By setting clear intentions for energy cleansing and protection, we create a conscious shift in our energy field. Simply affirming statements such as "I release all that no longer serves me" or "I am surrounded by a protective shield of light" can have a profound effect on our energetic state.

8. Boundaries and Self-Care: Establishing healthy energetic boundaries and practicing self-care play a vital role in energy protection. Setting limits, saying no when needed, and prioritizing activities that nourish your energy help maintain your energetic well-being. Taking regular breaks, engaging in activities that bring joy, and surrounding

Enhancing your personal energy levels

Energy is the life force that propels us forward, fuels our actions, and influences our overall well-being. Personal energy levels play a crucial role in our ability to thrive, accomplish goals, and maintain a sense of vitality. Energy medicine offers practical approaches to enhance and optimize our personal energy, enabling us to lead more fulfilling and balanced lives. Below we will explore the concept of personal energy, the principles behind energy medicine, and practical techniques to enhance and sustain our energy levels.

Personal energy refers to the dynamic and subtle force that animates our physical, mental, and emotional states. It encompasses our vitality, focus, emotional resilience, and overall zest for life. When our personal energy is high and balanced, we experience increased motivation, mental clarity, emotional stability, and a greater capacity to handle stress.

Energy medicine recognizes that personal energy is influenced by various factors, both internal and external. These factors include our thoughts, emotions, lifestyle choices, relationships, nutrition, physical activity, and the environment in which we live. By understanding and consciously managing these factors, we can enhance and maintain our personal energy levels.

Several techniques can assist in enhancing personal energy:

2. Conscious Breathwork: Deep and conscious breathing techniques, such as diaphragmatic breathing or alternate nostril breathing, help oxygenate the body, improve circulation, and enhance energy levels. By bringing awareness to the breath and engaging in regular breathwork practices, we can increase vitality and support overall well-being.

3. Mindful Movement: Engaging in physical activities that promote body awareness and mindfulness, such as yoga, tai chi, or dance, can invigorate personal energy. These practices combine conscious movement, breath

control, and focused attention, supporting the flow of energy throughout the body.

4. Restorative Sleep: Quality sleep is crucial for replenishing personal energy levels. Creating a sleep routine, maintaining a comfortable sleep environment, and practicing relaxation techniques before bed can enhance the depth and restorative nature of our sleep, leaving us feeling rejuvenated and energized upon waking.

5. Nutrition and Hydration: Fueling the body with nutrient-dense foods and staying properly hydrated are essential for optimal energy levels. A balanced diet rich in whole foods, including fruits, vegetables, whole grains, and lean proteins, provides the necessary nutrients for energy production. Drinking an adequate amount of water helps maintain hydration and supports cellular function.

6. Stress Management: Chronic stress can deplete personal energy levels. Incorporating stress management techniques, such as mindfulness meditation, journaling, or engaging in hobbies, helps reduce stress and cultivate emotional resilience. By actively managing stress, we conserve and replenish our personal energy.

7. Energetic Self-Care: Engaging in practices that nourish our energy field is essential for maintaining personal energy levels. This can include activities such as energy healing sessions, self-Reiki, or practicing self-care rituals that promote relaxation and energetic balance. Taking time to recharge and rebalance our energy is vital for sustained vitality.

8. Emotional Well-Being: Emotions have a profound impact on personal energy. Practicing emotional awareness, engaging in techniques like Emotional Freedom Techniques (EFT) or journaling, and seeking support from loved ones or professionals when needed can assist in managing emotions and preserving personal energy.

9. Energetic Boundaries: Establishing healthy energetic boundaries supports personal energy management. This involves setting limits, saying no when necessary, and honoring our own needs and priorities. Maintaining healthy boundaries helps conserve and protect our energy from unnecessary depletion.

10. Nature Connection: Spending time in nature rejuvenates personal energy. Engaging in activities such as walking in the park, hiking, or simply sitting under a tree allows us to recharge and reconnect with

Chapter Nine

Energy Medicine and Spirituality

Energy medicine and spirituality are two interconnected realms that offer profound insights into the nature of existence and the human experience. While energy medicine focuses on the subtle energies that flow within and around us, spirituality delves into the realms of the sacred and the transcendental. Below we will explore the relationship between energy medicine and spirituality, highlighting the connections, commonalities, and their potential synergy in facilitating healing and personal transformation.

Energy medicine recognizes that the human body is not merely a physical entity but also an intricate network of energy systems. It acknowledges the existence of subtle energies, such as life force energy, chi, or prana, which underlie and influence our physical, mental, and emotional well-being. Energy medicine techniques, such as Reiki, Healing Touch, and acupuncture, work with these subtle energies to restore balance and promote healing.

Spirituality, on the other hand, encompasses a broader understanding of the human experience, transcending the boundaries of the physical realm. It explores the nature of consciousness, the search for meaning and purpose, and the connection to something greater than ourselves. Spirituality often involves practices such as meditation, prayer, contemplation, and engagement with religious or philosophical traditions.

At their core, both energy medicine and spirituality recognize the existence of a profound interplay between energy and the sacred. Here are some ways in which energy medicine and spirituality intersect:

2. Holistic View of Health: Both energy medicine and spirituality embrace a holistic perspective of health, recognizing that well-being encompasses more than just the physical body. They acknowledge the interconnectedness of mind, body, and spirit and emphasize the importance of nurturing all aspects of our being to achieve optimal health.

3. Awareness of Subtle Energies: Energy medicine and spirituality acknowledge the presence and significance of subtle energies that influence our well-being. Energy medicine techniques work directly with these energies to restore balance, while spirituality invites us to attune our awareness to the subtle energies that permeate our existence and connect us to the divine.

4. Intention and Consciousness: Both energy medicine and spirituality recognize the power of intention and consciousness in shaping our reality. Energy medicine techniques involve setting intentions and directing healing energy, while spirituality emphasizes the role of conscious awareness, mindfulness, and focused intention in spiritual growth and personal transformation.

5. Connection to Something Greater: Energy medicine and spirituality recognize that human beings are part of a larger cosmic tapestry. Energy medicine practitioners often describe their work as channeling or being a conduit for healing energy, while spirituality acknowledges the presence of a divine or transcendent force that animates and sustains all of creation.

6. Transpersonal Experiences: Energy medicine and spirituality encompass experiences that go beyond the individual egoic self. Energy medicine practitioners often report feeling connected to a larger field of conscious-

ness or experiencing states of expanded awareness during healing sessions. Spirituality explores mystical experiences, transcendence, and a sense of unity with the divine and all of creation.

7. Personal Transformation and Healing: Both energy medicine and spirituality offer pathways for personal transformation and healing. Energy medicine techniques aim to restore balance, clear blockages, and promote well-being. Spirituality invites individuals to embark on a journey of self-discovery, inner growth, and alignment with their higher purpose.

The synergy between energy medicine and spirituality can enhance the transformative potential of both realms. By integrating energy medicine techniques with spiritual practices, individuals can cultivate a deeper connection to the sacred while facilitating healing and personal growth. For example, incorporating meditation or prayer into energy healing sessions can deepen the sense of presence and attunement to the divine energies being channeled.

It is important to note that while energy medicine and spirituality complement each other, they are not synonymous. Energy medicine encompasses a range of techniques and modalities,

The connection between energy medicine and spiritual growth

Energy medicine and spiritual growth are two interwoven paths that offer individuals a profound opportunity for personal transformation, self-discovery, and holistic well-being. While energy medicine focuses on the subtle energies that permeate our being, spiritual growth encompasses the expansion of consciousness, connection to the divine, and the unfolding of one's spiritual potential. Below we will explore the connection between energy medicine and spiritual growth, highlighting how they complement and support each other in facilitating the journey towards wholeness and inner awakening.

Energy medicine recognizes that the human body is not solely a physical entity but a complex network of energetic systems. It acknowledges the existence of subtle energies that flow within and around us, influencing our health and well-being. Energy medicine modalities, such as Reiki, Healing Touch, and acupuncture, work with these subtle energies to restore balance, clear blockages, and promote healing on physical, emotional, and spiritual levels.

Spiritual growth, on the other hand, involves the expansion of consciousness and the deepening of one's connection to the divine or higher aspects of existence. It encompasses the exploration of personal beliefs, values, and the search for meaning and purpose. Spiritual growth often involves practices such as meditation, prayer, mindfulness, contemplation, and engagement with religious or philosophical traditions.

The connection between energy medicine and spiritual growth arises from their shared understanding of the fundamental nature of existence and the interplay between energy and consciousness. Here are some ways in which energy medicine and spiritual growth intersect:

2. Awareness of Subtle Energies: Both energy medicine and spiritual growth acknowledge the presence and significance of subtle energies that permeate our being. Energy medicine techniques work directly with these energies, while spiritual practices invite individuals to attune their awareness to the subtle energies that underlie and connect all of creation.

3. Balance and Alignment: Energy medicine recognizes that imbalances or blockages in the energy system can lead to physical, emotional, and spiritual disharmony. By restoring balance and promoting the flow of en-

ergy, energy medicine techniques support the alignment of the individual's energy field, facilitating spiritual growth and well-being.

4. Clearing and Releasing: Energy medicine practices offer methods for clearing and releasing stagnant or negative energy from the energy field. This clearing process can extend beyond the physical body to include emotional and spiritual aspects, supporting the individual in letting go of limiting beliefs, unresolved emotions, and energetic attachments that impede spiritual growth.

5. Energetic Attunement: Energy medicine techniques, such as Reiki and Healing Touch, involve the transmission of healing energy from practitioner to recipient. These energetic transmissions can facilitate a deep sense of connection, peace, and relaxation, creating a fertile ground for spiritual growth and self-discovery.

6. Enhancing Intuition and Inner Wisdom: Energy medicine practices cultivate the development of intuitive abilities and the connection to one's inner wisdom. As individuals engage with their energy field and the subtle sensations and messages it provides, they develop a heightened sensitivity to their own needs, desires, and spiritual guidance.

7. Awakening Consciousness: Energy medicine and spiritual growth both support the expansion of consciousness. Energy medicine practices can facilitate shifts in awareness, allowing individuals to tap into deeper levels of consciousness and access expanded states of being. These shifts can catalyze spiritual growth by opening doors to new insights, understanding, and self-realization.

8. Integration of Body, Mind, and Spirit: Both energy medicine and spiritual growth recognize the importance of integrating the different aspects of the self - body, mind, and spirit. Energy medicine techniques work holistically, addressing the interconnected nature of these dimensions. Spiritual

growth encourages individuals to embrace the wholeness of their being and honor the interconnectedness of their physical, emotional, and

Kundalini energy and spiritual awakening

Kundalini energy, often described as the dormant cosmic energy coiled at the base of the spine, is a profound force that holds immense transformative potential. Its awakening is believed to initiate a journey of spiritual growth, self-realization, and expanded consciousness. Rooted in the ancient wisdom of yoga and energy medicine, Kundalini energy and its connection to spiritual awakening have captivated the interest of seekers throughout the ages. Below we will explore the concept of Kundalini energy, its role in spiritual awakening, and its relationship to energy medicine.

Kundalini, derived from the Sanskrit word meaning "coiled serpent," is said to reside in the subtle energy body, specifically in the energy center known as the Muladhara or root chakra. It represents the untapped potential and life force energy within each individual. Kundalini energy is likened to a dormant serpent awaiting awakening, and when activated, it ascends through the energy channels, known as nadis, along the spine, ultimately reaching the crown of the head, the Sahasrara or crown chakra.

The awakening of Kundalini energy is considered a profound spiritual event that can lead to spiritual growth, self-realization, and expanded consciousness. It is often described as a process of purification and transformation, as the rising energy clears energetic blockages, dissolves limitations, and awakens dormant faculties within the individual. Kundalini awakening is believed to bring about a heightened state of awareness, deepened spiritual experiences, and a profound sense of interconnectedness with all of creation.

Energy medicine approaches recognize Kundalini energy as a vital aspect of the human energy system. While energy medicine encompasses various techniques and modalities, Kundalini energy holds a unique place due to its transformative nature. Here are some aspects of Kundalini energy and its relationship to energy medicine:

2. Energy Activation and Flow: Kundalini awakening involves the activation and release of powerful energy within the individual. Energy medicine practices, such as breathwork, meditation, Reiki, and yoga, facilitate the activation and flow of energy throughout the body, supporting the awakening and harmonious ascent of Kundalini energy.

3. Energetic Clearing and Purification: Kundalini awakening is often accompanied by intense energetic experiences as the energy encounters and clears blockages and stagnant patterns within the individual's energy system. Energy medicine techniques can assist in clearing and purifying the energy field, facilitating a smoother and more balanced Kundalini awakening process.

4. Chakra Balancing and Alignment: The awakening of Kundalini energy involves the activation and harmonization of the chakra system. Energy medicine modalities, such as chakra balancing, assist in aligning and balancing the individual's energy centers, ensuring a smooth flow of Kundalini energy through the central energy channel, the Sushumna.

5. Energetic Grounding and Integration: Kundalini awakening can be a profound and intense experience, often accompanied by heightened states of consciousness. Energy medicine practices, including grounding techniques, help individuals remain anchored and integrated during this transformative process, ensuring that the awakened Kundalini energy is effectively integrated into daily life.

6. Healing and Transformation: Kundalini awakening is believed to catalyze deep healing and transformation on all levels of the individual's being. Energy medicine techniques support this healing process by addressing energetic imbalances, promoting self-awareness, and facilitating the release of past traumas and limiting beliefs that may hinder the individual's spiritual growth.

7. Consciousness Expansion and Spiritual Insights: Kundalini awakening can lead to expanded states of consciousness, opening doors to higher realms of perception and spiritual insights. Energy medicine practices, such as

Developing intuition and psychic abilities

Intuition and psychic abilities are innate human capacities that allow individuals to access information beyond the scope of ordinary perception. These extraordinary faculties provide a deeper understanding of the self, others, and the world around us. Rooted in the realm of energy medicine, the development of intuition and psychic abilities holds the potential for personal growth, spiritual exploration, and expanded consciousness. Below we will explore the nature of intuition and psychic abilities, their relationship to energy medicine, and practical techniques for their development.

Intuition can be understood as the direct knowing or understanding of something without the need for conscious reasoning or analysis. It is often described as a gut feeling, a hunch, or an inner knowing. Psychic abilities, on the other hand, refer to the broader range of extrasensory perceptions, including clairvoyance (clear seeing), clairaudience (clear hearing), clairsentience (clear sensing), and telepathy (mind-to-mind communication). These abilities allow individuals to access information beyond the limitations of the five physical senses.

Energy medicine recognizes that intuition and psychic abilities are closely linked to the subtle energies that permeate our being. Our energy field, or aura, is believed to contain information and impressions that can be accessed through heightened awareness and sensitivity. By understanding and working with these energies, individuals can cultivate and enhance their intuitive and psychic capacities.

Here are some key elements of developing intuition and psychic abilities within the realm of energy medicine:

2. Energetic Sensitivity: Developing intuition and psychic abilities requires the cultivation of energetic sensitivity. Energy medicine practices, such as meditation, breathwork, and Reiki, help individuals attune their awareness to subtle energetic sensations, allowing them to perceive and interpret energetic information.

3. Chakra Awareness: The chakra system, consisting of seven main energy centers along the central axis of the body, plays a vital role in intuition and psychic development. Each chakra is associated with specific qualities and functions. Energy medicine techniques, such as chakra balancing and clearing, support the harmonious functioning of the chakra system, facilitating the flow of intuitive and psychic energy.

4. Inner Listening: Developing intuition involves cultivating the ability to listen to the subtle whispers of our inner guidance. Energy medicine practices, such as mindfulness meditation and deep relaxation, create a space for inner stillness and receptive awareness. In this state, individuals can attune to their inner wisdom and receive intuitive insights.

5. Energetic Protection: As individuals open themselves to intuitive and psychic experiences, it is essential to establish energetic protection. Energy medicine techniques, such as visualizations, intention setting, and the use

of protective crystals, help create a safe and supportive energetic boundary, preventing unwanted influences or energy drains.

6. Developing the Clair Senses: Psychic abilities often involve the development of the clair senses, such as clairvoyance, clairaudience, and clairsentience. Energy medicine practices, such as guided imagery, energy scanning, and working with symbolic imagery, can help enhance and refine these psychic perceptions.

7. Healing and Clearing: Clearing personal energy blockages and resolving emotional wounds is vital for developing intuition and psychic abilities. Energy medicine techniques, including energy healing sessions, EFT (Emotional Freedom Techniques), and shadow work, support the release of energetic imprints that may hinder intuitive perceptions.

8. Trust and Practice: Developing intuition and psychic abilities requires trust in one's inner wisdom and continuous practice. By engaging in regular meditation, journaling, energy healing exercises, and working with divination tools, individuals can strengthen their intuitive connections and deepen their psychic awareness.

9. Ethical Considerations: It is essential to approach the development of intuition and psychic abilities with integrity and ethical

Chapter Ten

The Future of Energy Medicine

Energy medicine is an evolving field that has gained recognition and popularity in recent years as a holistic approach to healthcare and well-being. With its emphasis on the interplay between energy, consciousness, and the physical body, energy medicine offers a unique perspective on healing and personal transformation. As we move forward into the future, energy medicine holds the potential to revolutionize healthcare, expand our understanding of human potential, and create a more integrated approach to well-being. Below we will explore the future of energy medicine, including emerging trends, advancements, and the transformative impact it may have on individuals and society as a whole.

2. Integration of Conventional and Energy Medicine: The future of energy medicine lies in the integration of conventional medical practices with energy-based modalities. As research continues to validate the efficacy of energy medicine techniques, we can expect to see greater collaboration between conventional healthcare providers and energy medicine practitioners. This integration will offer patients a more comprehensive and personalized approach to healing, addressing the physical, emotional, mental, and energetic aspects of their well-being.

3. Scientific Validation: While energy medicine has been met with some skepticism in the past, ongoing scientific research is beginning to provide empirical evidence for its effectiveness. As technology advances, we can expect more sophisticated methods to study and measure the subtle en-

ergies and their impact on health and healing. This scientific validation will further establish energy medicine as a credible and evidence-based approach to healthcare.

4. Personalized Medicine: Energy medicine recognizes the uniqueness of each individual's energy system and the importance of personalized approaches to healing. In the future, we can anticipate the development of technologies and diagnostic tools that assess an individual's energy field and provide tailored recommendations for energy balancing and healing. This shift towards personalized medicine will empower individuals to take an active role in their own healing journey.

5. Technological Innovations: Technology will play a significant role in the future of energy medicine. Advancements in biofeedback devices, wearable sensors, and virtual reality applications will allow individuals to monitor and interact with their energy field in real-time. These technologies will facilitate self-care practices, energy balancing, and provide individuals with a deeper understanding of their energetic state.

6. Mind-Body Integration: Energy medicine recognizes the profound interconnection between the mind, body, and spirit. In the future, we can expect to see a greater emphasis on mind-body integration within healthcare systems. This integration will involve the incorporation of energy medicine techniques, such as breathwork, meditation, and energy healing, alongside traditional medical interventions. By addressing the underlying energetic imbalances and promoting self-awareness, mind-body integration will foster a more holistic approach to healing and well-being.

7. Energy Medicine in Preventive Care: The future of healthcare will shift towards a greater focus on preventive care. Energy medicine offers valuable tools for maintaining optimal health and preventing disease by addressing energetic imbalances before they manifest as physical symptoms. By

incorporating energy medicine practices into preventive care programs, individuals can take proactive steps to maintain their energetic well-being and overall health.

8. Global Adoption: Energy medicine is gaining recognition and acceptance worldwide. As awareness spreads and people experience the benefits of energy medicine firsthand, we can anticipate a global shift towards incorporating energy-based practices into healthcare systems. This will lead to increased accessibility and integration of energy medicine techniques in various cultural and geographical contexts.

9. Holistic Education: The future of energy medicine will involve the integration of energy-based practices into conventional medical and healthcare education. Medical schools, nursing programs, and allied health professions will incorporate courses on energy medicine, energy anatomy, and integrative approaches to healing. This educational shift will empower healthcare professionals to incorporate energy medicine techniques into their practice and offer more comprehensive care to their patients.

Integrating energy medicine into mainstream healthcare

Energy medicine, with its focus on the subtle energy systems that influence our health and well-being, has emerged as a valuable complement to mainstream healthcare practices. While it has gained popularity among alternative and holistic health enthusiasts, the integration of energy medicine into mainstream healthcare has been a gradual process. However, as scientific research continues to shed light on the effectiveness of energy-based approaches, there is a growing recognition of the potential benefits that energy medicine can offer in enhancing patient care and promoting holistic healing. Below we will explore the integration of energy medicine into mainstream healthcare, its benefits, challenges, and the transformative impact it can have on healthcare systems.

2. Evidence-Based Research: The integration of energy medicine into mainstream healthcare requires a strong foundation of evidence-based research. As more studies are conducted on energy medicine techniques, such as Reiki, Healing Touch, and acupuncture, there is a growing body of evidence supporting their effectiveness in improving patient outcomes. Rigorous scientific research helps bridge the gap between anecdotal evidence and mainstream acceptance, providing healthcare practitioners with the confidence to incorporate energy medicine into their practice.

3. Holistic Approach to Healing: Energy medicine embraces a holistic approach to healing, recognizing the interconnectedness of the mind, body, and spirit. By integrating energy medicine techniques into mainstream healthcare, practitioners can address not only the physical symptoms but also the underlying energetic imbalances that may contribute to illness. This holistic perspective allows for a more comprehensive and patient-centered approach to healthcare.

4. Complementary Therapies: Energy medicine can complement conventional medical treatments by enhancing their effectiveness and supporting the healing process. For example, energy-based techniques can help alleviate pain, reduce stress and anxiety, improve sleep, and enhance overall well-being. Integrating energy medicine into mainstream healthcare allows for a wider range of therapeutic options, providing patients with a more personalized and integrated approach to their care.

5. Patient Empowerment: Energy medicine empowers patients to take an active role in their healing journey. By incorporating energy medicine practices into mainstream healthcare, patients gain access to self-care techniques, such as mindfulness, breathwork, and energy balancing exercises. These practices promote self-awareness, stress reduction, and overall well-being, allowing patients to actively participate in their own healing process.

6. Preventive Care: Energy medicine's emphasis on maintaining energetic balance and promoting wellness aligns with the growing focus on preventive care in healthcare systems. By integrating energy medicine into mainstream healthcare, practitioners can educate patients about energy management, stress reduction techniques, and healthy lifestyle choices that support optimal well-being. This preventive approach can help reduce the incidence of chronic diseases and improve overall health outcomes.

7. Collaborative Care: The integration of energy medicine into mainstream healthcare encourages collaborative care models where healthcare practitioners from different disciplines work together to provide comprehensive and holistic care to patients. This interdisciplinary approach fosters communication, cooperation, and the exchange of knowledge, ultimately benefiting the patient's overall health and well-being.

8. Training and Education: To facilitate the integration of energy medicine into mainstream healthcare, it is crucial to provide healthcare practitioners with adequate training and education in energy-based approaches. Integrative medicine programs, continuing education courses, and workshops can equip healthcare professionals with the knowledge and skills necessary to incorporate energy medicine techniques into their practice. By expanding training opportunities, healthcare systems can nurture a generation of practitioners who are adept in both conventional and energy-based healing modalities.

9. Research Integration Centers: The establishment of research integration centers can serve as hubs for studying the efficacy and safety of energy medicine techniques. These centers can collaborate with academic institutions, healthcare organizations, and funding agencies to conduct rigorous research, collect data, and disseminate findings. Such collaborative efforts will not only contribute to the evidence base of energy medicine but also

Innovations in energy medicine research and technology

Energy medicine, with its focus on the subtle energies that underlie our physical, mental, and emotional well-being, has witnessed remarkable advancements in research and technology in recent years. As our understanding of energy and its impact on health deepens, scientists and practitioners are exploring innovative approaches to further unlock the healing potential of energy medicine. Below we will explore the latest innovations in energy medicine research and technology, highlighting their impact on healthcare, well-being, and the future of holistic healing.

2. Biofield Imaging: The development of advanced imaging technologies has revolutionized the study of the human biofield, a subtle energy field that surrounds and permeates the body. Biofield imaging techniques, such as gas discharge visualization (GDV) and bioelectrography, capture real-time images of the energy field, providing insights into its dynamics and patterns. These technologies enable researchers to study the effects of energy medicine interventions and track changes in the biofield before and after treatment.

3. Electrophysiological Measurements: Researchers are utilizing sophisticated electrophysiological measurement devices to study the effects of energy medicine on the body's electrical activity. Techniques such as electroencephalography (EEG) and heart rate variability (HRV) analysis help assess changes in brainwave patterns, heart rate, and autonomic nervous system function before, during, and after energy medicine interventions. These measurements provide objective data on the physiological effects of energy medicine techniques.

4. Quantum Biology: The field of quantum biology explores the intersection of quantum physics and biology, investigating how quantum phenomena influence biological processes. Researchers are studying the role of

quantum coherence and entanglement in cellular communication and signaling, shedding light on the mechanisms underlying energy-based healing modalities. Understanding the quantum aspects of energy medicine may lead to the development of more targeted and effective interventions.

5. Wearable Technology: The rise of wearable technology has opened new avenues for monitoring and enhancing personal energy and well-being. Devices such as biofeedback sensors, smart jewelry, and smart clothing can measure various physiological parameters, such as heart rate, skin conductance, and respiratory rate, providing real-time feedback on the individual's energy state. These wearable devices allow individuals to track their energy levels, manage stress, and make informed lifestyle choices to optimize their well-being.

6. Remote Healing and Telemedicine: The advent of telecommunication technology has enabled remote energy healing and telemedicine practices. Energy medicine practitioners can remotely transmit healing energy and provide guidance to individuals in need, regardless of geographical distance. Telemedicine platforms facilitate virtual consultations, enabling healthcare professionals to incorporate energy medicine techniques into their practice and reach a wider range of patients.

7. Artificial Intelligence and Machine Learning: The integration of artificial intelligence (AI) and machine learning algorithms in energy medicine research has the potential to revolutionize diagnosis, treatment, and personalized healthcare. AI can analyze large datasets of energy medicine research, identify patterns, and provide insights into the efficacy of different interventions. Machine learning algorithms can assist in developing personalized treatment plans based on individual energy profiles, optimizing therapeutic outcomes.

8. Bioinformatics and Data Analysis: With the proliferation of energy medicine research, bioinformatics and data analysis techniques are becoming essential tools for understanding complex energy systems. Researchers are utilizing computational models, network analysis, and data mining techniques to decipher the intricate relationships within the energy field, identify biomarkers of health and disease, and develop predictive models for energy-based interventions.

9. Energy Medicine Apps and Platforms: Mobile applications and online platforms are emerging as accessible resources for energy medicine practice and education. Energy medicine apps provide guided meditations, breathing exercises, and energy balancing techniques that individuals can practice at their convenience. Online platforms offer courses, webinars, and communities for sharing knowledge and experiences

The ethical considerations and challenges of energy medicine

Energy medicine, with its focus on the subtle energies that influence health and well-being, offers a unique approach to healing and personal transformation. As the field continues to gain recognition and popularity, it is crucial to explore the ethical considerations and challenges that arise in the practice of energy medicine. With its holistic and often self-directed nature, energy medicine presents a distinctive set of ethical dilemmas that practitioners and recipients must navigate. Below we will delve into the ethical considerations and challenges of energy medicine, shedding light on the boundaries, responsibilities, and potential risks involved.

2. Informed Consent: In energy medicine, it is essential to obtain informed consent from individuals seeking treatment. Practitioners should clearly explain the nature of the energy medicine techniques, potential

benefits, and any possible risks or side effects. Informed consent ensures that recipients are aware of the nature of the intervention and can make autonomous decisions about their care.

3. Scope of Practice: Ethical considerations arise regarding the scope of practice in energy medicine. Practitioners should be knowledgeable about their own limitations and refer clients to appropriate healthcare professionals when necessary. Recognizing the boundaries of their expertise ensures the well-being and safety of recipients and promotes collaboration within the healthcare system.

4. Professional Competence and Training: Ethical practice in energy medicine requires practitioners to maintain professional competence through ongoing education and training. It is crucial to ensure that practitioners have the necessary knowledge, skills, and experience to provide safe and effective energy medicine interventions. Continuing education and professional development support ethical practice by keeping practitioners up-to-date with advancements and best practices in the field.

5. Client Confidentiality and Privacy: Like any healthcare practice, energy medicine requires practitioners to uphold client confidentiality and privacy. Practitioners should respect the confidential nature of the information shared during sessions and take appropriate measures to safeguard client privacy. Maintaining confidentiality builds trust and establishes a safe space for clients to share their experiences.

6. Cultural Sensitivity and Respect: Energy medicine encompasses diverse cultural, spiritual, and belief systems. Practitioners must approach their work with cultural sensitivity, respect, and open-mindedness. It is crucial to honor and acknowledge the diversity of clients' beliefs, values, and traditions, and to refrain from imposing personal beliefs or making claims that contradict an individual's cultural or religious background.

7. Financial Transparency: Ethical practice in energy medicine requires practitioners to be transparent about their fees and financial arrangements. Clear communication regarding the costs of services, payment methods, and refund policies ensures that clients are well-informed and can make financial decisions based on accurate information.

8. Vulnerable Populations: Practitioners of energy medicine should be mindful of the vulnerability of certain populations, such as children, the elderly, and individuals with cognitive or psychological impairments. Extra care should be taken to obtain informed consent, provide appropriate explanations, and ensure the well-being of vulnerable recipients. Practitioners should be cautious about making claims or promises that exploit the vulnerability of individuals seeking help.

9. Ethical Marketing and Advertising: Practitioners in energy medicine should adhere to ethical guidelines when marketing their services. Claims and advertisements should be truthful, accurate, and not misleading. Practitioners should avoid making unfounded claims about their abilities or the effectiveness of energy medicine techniques, respecting the boundaries of scientific evidence and maintaining integrity in their promotional activities.

10. Maintaining Professional Boundaries: Establishing and maintaining professional boundaries is essential in energy medicine. Practitioners should establish clear guidelines regarding physical touch, appropriate behavior, and professional-client relationships. Practitioners must be aware of the potential for transference and countertransference, maintaining a therapeutic and objective perspective.

11. Emergency Preparedness: Ethical practice in energy medicine requires practitioners to be

Chapter Eleven

Energy Medicine for Stress and Anxiety

In today's fast-paced world, stress and anxiety have become prevalent challenges that affect millions of individuals worldwide. While conventional approaches to managing stress and anxiety are widely available, energy medicine offers a unique and holistic perspective on addressing these conditions. By working with the subtle energies that permeate our bodies and influence our well-being, energy medicine provides effective tools and techniques for finding inner balance, promoting relaxation, and alleviating the symptoms of stress and anxiety. Below we will explore the application of energy medicine in the context of stress and anxiety, shedding light on its benefits, techniques, and its potential to enhance overall well-being.

2. Understanding Stress and Anxiety: Stress is the body's response to external pressures, while anxiety is a psychological response characterized by excessive worry and apprehension. Both stress and anxiety can have profound effects on our physical, mental, and emotional well-being. Energy medicine recognizes that stress and anxiety not only affect our thoughts and emotions but also disrupt the subtle energy systems within our bodies.

3. Energetic Imbalances and Blockages: Energy medicine views stress and anxiety as manifestations of energetic imbalances and blockages within our energy field. These imbalances can disrupt the smooth flow of energy, leading to physical and emotional discomfort. By identifying and address-

ing these energetic imbalances, energy medicine techniques aim to restore harmony and balance within the individual's energy system.

4. Breathwork and Grounding: Breathwork is a fundamental energy medicine technique that can be highly effective in managing stress and anxiety. Conscious, deep breathing techniques activate the body's relaxation response, promoting a state of calm and reducing stress hormones. Grounding exercises, such as visualizations and mindful awareness of the body, help individuals reconnect with the present moment and anchor their energy, alleviating feelings of anxiety and promoting a sense of stability.

5. Energy Balancing Techniques: Energy medicine offers various techniques for balancing and harmonizing the energy system. Modalities such as Reiki, Healing Touch, and acupuncture work to clear blockages, release stagnant energy, and restore the flow of vital life force energy. These techniques facilitate relaxation, support the body's natural healing abilities, and reduce the physical and emotional symptoms associated with stress and anxiety.

6. EFT (Emotional Freedom Techniques): EFT, also known as tapping, is an energy psychology technique that combines acupressure points with cognitive and emotional processing. By tapping on specific meridian points while focusing on the stress or anxiety-inducing issue, EFT can help release emotional and energetic blockages, promoting a sense of calm and relaxation. EFT is known for its quick effectiveness and can be easily learned and practiced by individuals as a self-help tool.

7. Mindfulness and Meditation: Mindfulness and meditation practices are integral to energy medicine approaches for stress and anxiety. These practices cultivate present-moment awareness, helping individuals observe and detach from anxious thoughts and worries. By focusing on the breath, sensations, or a specific object of meditation, individuals can develop re-

silience, improve emotional regulation, and experience a greater sense of inner calm and well-being.

8. Vibrational Medicine: Vibrational medicine involves the use of specific frequencies, sounds, and vibrations to promote healing and balance. Sound therapy, such as using singing bowls, tuning forks, or listening to calming music, can induce a state of relaxation, reduce stress, and restore energetic harmony. Additionally, gemstone therapy, aromatherapy, and flower essences are used in energy medicine to support emotional well-being and energetic balance.

9. Self-Care Practices: Energy medicine emphasizes the importance of self-care practices in managing stress and anxiety. Engaging in activities such as regular exercise, healthy nutrition, quality sleep, and nurturing self-care rituals can help

Breathing techniques for energy balance

Breath is the essence of life. It is an involuntary process that sustains us, but it can also be a powerful tool for enhancing our well-being and achieving energetic balance. In the realm of energy medicine, breathing techniques play a significant role in harmonizing and balancing our subtle energies, facilitating relaxation, and promoting overall health and vitality. Below we will explore the relationship between breath and energy balance, and delve into various breathing techniques used in energy medicine for optimal well-being.

2. The Breath-Energy Connection: Energy medicine recognizes that breath is intimately connected to our subtle energy systems. Each breath we take influences the flow of vital life force energy within us. When we breathe consciously and with intention, we can positively impact our energy field, promoting balance and harmony.

3. Diaphragmatic Breathing: Diaphragmatic breathing, also known as belly breathing or deep breathing, is a foundational breathing technique used in energy medicine. By engaging the diaphragm muscle and expanding the abdomen on inhalation, we maximize the intake of oxygen and stimulate the relaxation response. Diaphragmatic breathing calms the nervous system, reduces stress hormones, and promotes a state of energetic balance and well-being.

4. Alternate Nostril Breathing: Alternate nostril breathing is a powerful technique for balancing the flow of energy within the body. By using the thumb and ring finger to alternately close and open the nostrils, this technique balances the left and right energy channels, known as nadis or meridians. Alternate nostril breathing enhances energetic harmony, clears blockages, and promotes mental clarity and emotional balance.

5. Ujjayi Breathing: Ujjayi breathing, also called "victorious breath," is a yogic breathing technique that balances and energizes the body and mind. It involves slightly constricting the throat during inhalation and exhalation, creating a gentle, oceanic sound. Ujjayi breathing enhances oxygenation, calms the mind, and supports energetic flow throughout the body, fostering a sense of groundedness and well-being.

6. Three-Part Breath: The three-part breath, also known as yogic complete breath or full yogic breath, engages the three primary areas of the lungs: the abdomen, diaphragm, and chest. This technique expands the capacity of the lungs and optimizes oxygen intake. By utilizing the full capacity of the breath, we enhance the flow of prana (life force energy) throughout the body, promoting vitality, relaxation, and energetic balance.

7. Box Breathing: Box breathing, also called square breathing or four-square breathing, is a simple yet effective technique for calming the mind and balancing energy. It involves inhaling, holding the breath, exhal-

ing, and holding the breath again, each for an equal duration. This pattern creates a square-like shape, hence the name. Box breathing regulates the nervous system, reduces stress, and brings about a state of energetic equilibrium.

8. Coherent Breathing: Coherent breathing, also known as resonant or heart-centered breathing, focuses on maintaining a consistent rhythm and balance between inhalation and exhalation. This technique synchronizes the breath with the heart rate, promoting heart coherence and balancing the autonomic nervous system. Coherent breathing fosters relaxation, reduces anxiety, and enhances overall energetic coherence and well-being.

9. Energizing Breath: Energizing breath techniques, such as Kapalabhati (skull shining breath) and Breath of Fire, are energizing and invigorating practices used in energy medicine. These rapid and forceful exhalations, combined with passive inhalations, stimulate the solar plexus chakra, energize the body, and clear stagnant

Energy medicine and relaxation response

In our fast-paced and stressful modern lives, finding ways to induce deep relaxation and restore balance is crucial for our well-being. While various techniques and practices exist, energy medicine offers a unique and powerful approach to achieving profound relaxation through the manipulation and balancing of subtle energies within the body. By working with the body's energy systems, energy medicine techniques can elicit the relaxation response, a state of deep calm and rejuvenation. Below we will explore the relationship between energy medicine and the relaxation response, shedding light on the benefits, techniques, and the potential for healing and transformation.

2. Understanding the Relaxation Response: The relaxation response is the body's natural antidote to stress and a state of deep relaxation that counters the effects of the stress response. When activated, the relaxation response triggers physiological changes, such as reduced heart rate, lowered blood pressure, and decreased muscle tension. It promotes a sense of calm, enhances mental clarity, and supports overall well-being.

3. Energy Medicine and Subtle Energies: Energy medicine recognizes that the human body is composed of intricate energetic systems that influence our physical, mental, and emotional well-being. These energy systems, including the meridians, chakras, and aura, play a vital role in our overall health and vitality. By understanding and working with these subtle energies, energy medicine techniques can facilitate the relaxation response and promote deep relaxation and healing.

4. Balancing Energy Flow: Energy medicine techniques aim to balance and optimize the flow of energy within the body. When the energy flow is harmonious and unobstructed, the body is better equipped to enter a state of deep relaxation. Practices such as Reiki, Healing Touch, and acupuncture work to clear energy blockages, release stagnant energy, and restore the natural flow of life force energy. By balancing the energy systems, these techniques support the body's ability to activate the relaxation response.

5. Breathwork and Energetic Balance: Breathwork is a fundamental aspect of energy medicine and plays a pivotal role in inducing the relaxation response. Conscious and intentional breathing techniques, such as diaphragmatic breathing and alternate nostril breathing, enhance oxygenation, stimulate the parasympathetic nervous system, and activate the relaxation response. These techniques synchronize the breath with the flow of subtle energy, promoting energetic balance and deep relaxation.

6. Energetic Healing Modalities: Energy medicine encompasses a variety of modalities that facilitate relaxation and activate the body's innate healing capacities. Techniques such as Reiki, Healing Touch, and Qi Gong work directly with the body's energy field, promoting relaxation, releasing tension, and facilitating energetic balance. These modalities can induce a deep sense of calm and relaxation, allowing the body to enter a state of optimal healing and rejuvenation.

7. Mind-Body Connection: Energy medicine recognizes the intimate connection between the mind and body. By addressing the energetic imbalances and blockages within the body, energy medicine techniques can influence the mind and emotions, promoting a state of deep relaxation. The mind-body connection plays a significant role in the relaxation response, and energy medicine practices leverage this connection to support relaxation and healing.

8. Visualization and Guided Imagery: Visualization and guided imagery are powerful tools used in energy medicine to promote relaxation and activate the relaxation response. By utilizing the power of the mind's imagery, individuals can create mental images of peaceful and tranquil environments, invoking a sense of relaxation and well-being. These practices engage the creative and subconscious mind, facilitating the relaxation response and deepening the relaxation experience.

9. Meditation and Mindfulness: Meditation and mindfulness practices are integral to energy medicine and play a crucial role in inducing the relaxation response. These practices involve focusing the attention on the present

Energy medicine for emotional resilience

Emotional resilience is the ability to adapt, bounce back, and maintain a sense of well-being in the face of adversity or stressful situations. In today's fast-paced world, where emotional challenges are prevalent, cultivating emotional resilience is essential for our overall mental and emotional health. Energy medicine offers valuable tools and techniques to support emotional resilience by working with the body's subtle energy systems. By harnessing and balancing these energies, individuals can enhance their ability to navigate emotions, regulate stress, and cultivate inner strength. Below we will explore the relationship between energy medicine and emotional resilience, uncovering the benefits, techniques, and transformative potential for well-being.

2. Understanding Emotional Resilience: Emotional resilience is the capacity to adapt and maintain equilibrium in the face of life's challenges, stressors, and emotional experiences. It involves recognizing and managing emotions effectively, developing healthy coping strategies, and fostering a sense of inner strength and balance. Energy medicine offers unique perspectives and techniques to support emotional resilience by addressing the energetic aspects of emotional well-being.

3. Subtle Energy Systems and Emotions: Energy medicine recognizes that emotions have an energetic component and are influenced by the body's subtle energy systems. Emotions are seen as patterns of energy that can either flow freely or become blocked and stagnant. By working with the body's energy systems, energy medicine techniques aim to balance and harmonize these energy patterns, promoting emotional well-being and resilience.

4. Emotional Release and Energy Clearing: Energy medicine techniques, such as Emotional Freedom Techniques (EFT), allow individuals to release emotional blockages and promote emotional resilience. EFT involves tapping on specific acupressure points while focusing on the emotion or

issue at hand. This process can help individuals acknowledge and process challenging emotions, release energy blockages, and promote emotional balance and resilience.

5. Chakra Balancing: The chakra system, a central aspect of energy medicine, is closely associated with emotions and emotional well-being. The seven main chakras are considered energy centers that influence different aspects of our physical, mental, and emotional states. Balancing and harmonizing the chakras through energy medicine techniques, such as visualization, intention, and energy healing, can support emotional resilience by promoting energetic balance and emotional well-being.

6. Mind-Body Techniques: Energy medicine incorporates mind-body techniques that can enhance emotional resilience. Practices such as mindfulness meditation, breathwork, and visualization help individuals develop present-moment awareness, regulate emotions, and cultivate a sense of inner calm and balance. These techniques enable individuals to observe and respond to emotions in a more balanced and resilient manner.

7. Self-Care and Energetic Maintenance: Energy medicine emphasizes self-care practices as essential for emotional resilience. Engaging in activities that promote self-nurturing, such as regular exercise, quality sleep, healthy nutrition, and time for relaxation and rejuvenation, supports energetic balance and emotional well-being. Self-care practices replenish and restore the body's energy, enhancing resilience in the face of emotional challenges.

8. Energetic Boundaries and Protection: Emotional resilience involves establishing healthy boundaries and protecting one's energetic space. Energy medicine techniques, such as visualization and intention, can be employed to create energetic boundaries that safeguard against emotional overload and promote a sense of inner stability. These techniques allow individuals

to manage their energy and protect themselves from external influences that may undermine emotional well-being.

9. Self-Reflection and Awareness: Energy medicine encourages self-reflection and increased self-awareness as vital components of emotional resilience. By cultivating a deeper understanding of one's emotions, triggers, and patterns, individuals can develop strategies to effectively respond to challenging emotions and build resilience. Self-reflection practices, such as journaling, meditation, or working with a therapist,

Chapter Twelve

Diet, Nutrition, and Energy Medicine

Diet and nutrition play a vital role in maintaining our physical health, but their impact goes beyond the realm of the physical. In the context of energy medicine, diet and nutrition are seen as crucial factors in supporting and optimizing the body's subtle energy systems. What we eat not only affects our physical vitality but also influences the flow of energy within our bodies. By understanding the relationship between diet, nutrition, and energy medicine, individuals can make conscious choices that nourish their subtle energies and promote overall well-being. Below we will explore the significance of diet and nutrition in energy medicine, uncovering the benefits, considerations, and practical strategies for harnessing the power of food to support optimal energetic balance.

2. The Connection between Food and Energy: Energy medicine recognizes that food carries vibrational energy that directly impacts our own energetic state. Different foods possess unique energetic qualities that can either enhance or hinder the flow of energy within our bodies. By choosing foods that resonate with our body's energetic needs, we can support the harmonious flow of subtle energies and promote overall well-being.

3. Whole Foods and Vitality: Energy medicine emphasizes the importance of consuming whole, minimally processed foods. Whole foods, such as fruits, vegetables, whole grains, and lean proteins, are rich in nutrients and life force energy. They provide the essential vitamins, minerals, and antioxidants necessary for maintaining the health and vitality of our subtle

energy systems. By prioritizing whole foods, we nourish our bodies at both the physical and energetic levels.

4. The Role of Macronutrients: Macronutrients, including carbohydrates, proteins, and fats, are essential components of our diet that provide the energy needed for optimal bodily functions. In energy medicine, balancing these macronutrients is important for supporting stable energy levels and overall energetic equilibrium. A balanced diet that includes appropriate portions of carbohydrates, high-quality proteins, and healthy fats promotes sustained energy and supports the body's energy systems.

5. Energetic Imbalances and Food Choices: Energy medicine recognizes that imbalances in our energy systems can manifest as cravings or aversions to certain foods. These preferences or aversions may indicate underlying energetic imbalances. By paying attention to our body's cues and observing our responses to different foods, we can identify potential energetic imbalances and make conscious dietary adjustments to restore harmony and balance.

6. Food Energetics and Traditional Healing Systems: Traditional healing systems, such as Ayurveda and Traditional Chinese Medicine, have long recognized the energetic qualities of food. These systems categorize foods based on their energetic properties, such as hot, cold, warming, cooling, and dampening. Understanding the energetics of food can guide us in selecting the appropriate foods to restore energetic balance and support specific health concerns.

7. Nutrient Density and Energy Systems: Nutrient-dense foods provide an abundance of vitamins, minerals, and phytochemicals that support the body's energy systems. Antioxidant-rich foods, such as berries, leafy greens, and nuts, help protect the body against oxidative stress and promote healthy energy flow. Consuming a diverse range of nutrient-dense

foods ensures that our energy systems receive the necessary support for optimal functioning.

8. Hydration and Energy Flow: Proper hydration is vital for maintaining the flow of energy within the body. Water acts as a conductor of energy and facilitates the movement of subtle energies throughout the body. Dehydration can lead to stagnation and imbalance in the energy systems. Drinking an adequate amount of water daily supports hydration and promotes the optimal flow of energy.

9. Mindful Eating and Energy Absorption: Energy medicine emphasizes the importance of mindful eating for optimizing energy absorption. Mindful eating involves being

Foods that support energy balance

Food is not only a source of sustenance but also a means to support the balance and flow of energy within our bodies. In the realm of energy medicine, certain foods are recognized for their ability to promote energetic balance and vitality. By incorporating these foods into our diet, we can optimize our overall well-being, enhance our energy levels, and support the harmonious functioning of our subtle energetic systems. Below we will explore a variety of foods that play a significant role in supporting energy balance, shedding light on their benefits, nutritional properties, and their impact on our energetic well-being.

2. Leafy Greens: Leafy greens, such as spinach, kale, and Swiss chard, are nutritional powerhouses that support energy balance. Packed with vitamins, minerals, and antioxidants, leafy greens provide essential nutrients for our cells and energy systems. They are also rich in chlorophyll, a pigment that helps cleanse and oxygenate the blood, promoting healthy energy flow and vitality.

3. Whole Grains: Whole grains, including quinoa, brown rice, and oats, are excellent sources of complex carbohydrates, fiber, and B vitamins. These nutrients provide sustained energy and help stabilize blood sugar levels, preventing energy spikes and crashes. Whole grains also contain minerals that support energy production and help maintain the integrity of our energetic systems.

4. Nuts and Seeds: Nuts and seeds, such as almonds, walnuts, flaxseeds, and chia seeds, are dense in nutrients and healthy fats. They provide a combination of protein, fiber, and essential fatty acids that support energy balance and help regulate blood sugar levels. Nuts and seeds are also a good source of magnesium, a mineral vital for energy production and the functioning of our energy systems.

5. Berries: Berries, such as blueberries, strawberries, and raspberries, are not only delicious but also rich in antioxidants and phytochemicals. These compounds protect our cells from oxidative stress and inflammation, supporting the overall health and vitality of our energy systems. Berries also provide a natural source of sweetness without causing drastic blood sugar fluctuations.

6. Citrus Fruits: Citrus fruits, including oranges, lemons, and grapefruits, are known for their high vitamin C content. Vitamin C is essential for the production of collagen, a protein that supports the integrity of our blood vessels and energy pathways. Citrus fruits also provide natural refreshment and hydration, which are vital for maintaining energy balance.

7. Fermented Foods: Fermented foods, such as sauerkraut, kimchi, and yogurt, are rich in beneficial bacteria known as probiotics. These friendly bacteria support gut health and digestion, which plays a crucial role in our overall energy balance. A healthy gut promotes optimal nutrient absorption and helps maintain the integrity of our energy systems.

8. Herbs and Spices: Herbs and spices, such as ginger, turmeric, cinnamon, and cayenne pepper, not only add flavor to our meals but also offer numerous health benefits. Many herbs and spices have antioxidant and anti-inflammatory properties, supporting overall well-being and energy balance. Additionally, some spices, like ginger and cayenne pepper, can help increase circulation and promote energy flow.

9. Dark Chocolate: Good news for chocolate lovers - dark chocolate (with a high percentage of cocoa) can support energy balance. Dark chocolate contains antioxidants, flavonoids, and magnesium, which contribute to its health-promoting properties. Enjoying a small piece of dark chocolate can provide a satisfying energy boost while offering a delightful treat.

10. Herbal Teas: Herbal teas, such as chamomile, peppermint, and ginseng

The impact of nutrition on the energy body

Nutrition plays a fundamental role in our physical health, but its impact extends beyond the physical body. In the realm of energy medicine, nutrition is recognized for its profound influence on the energy body—the intricate network of subtle energies that permeate and influence our overall well-being. The foods we consume directly impact the flow, balance, and vibrancy of these subtle energies. By understanding the relationship between nutrition and the energy body, we can make informed dietary choices that support our energetic well-being and promote optimal health. Below we will explore the impact of nutrition on the energy body, uncovering the benefits, considerations, and practical strategies for nurturing our subtle energies through conscious eating.

2. The Energy Body and Subtle Energies: Energy medicine views the human body as an interconnected system of subtle energies. These energies, including prana, chi, or life force energy, flow through channels or meridi-

ans, nourishing and sustaining the physical, mental, and emotional aspects of our being. Nutrition plays a critical role in supporting the vitality and balance of these subtle energies.

3. Energetic Qualities of Food: Energy medicine recognizes that each food carries its own unique energetic qualities. Foods can be classified as energetically warming, cooling, contracting, or expanding, based on their impact on the body's energy system. For example, spices like ginger or cayenne pepper have a warming and invigorating effect, while cucumbers or melons have a cooling and hydrating effect. Understanding the energetic qualities of food can help us make choices that support energetic balance.

4. Pranic Foods: Prana, a vital life force energy, is abundant in fresh, whole foods that are minimally processed and closest to their natural state. These pranic foods include fruits, vegetables, nuts, seeds, and sprouts. Pranic foods are rich in enzymes, vitamins, minerals, and antioxidants, which support the flow and vitality of the subtle energies. By prioritizing pranic foods, we provide our energy body with essential nutrients and life force energy.

5. Colorful Foods: The vibrancy and color of fruits and vegetables offer valuable insights into their energetic qualities. Foods with vibrant colors, such as berries, leafy greens, and oranges, are rich in antioxidants and phytochemicals. These compounds protect the energy body from oxidative stress and support its overall vitality. Including a variety of colorful foods in our diet ensures a diverse range of energetic nourishment.

6. Hydration and Energy Flow: Proper hydration is essential for the optimal flow of energy within the body. Water acts as a conduit for subtle energies, facilitating their movement and distribution throughout the energy body. Adequate hydration supports cellular function, detoxification, and

the overall balance of our energetic systems. Drinking pure, filtered water is crucial for maintaining hydration and supporting the energy body.

7. Gut Health and Energy Assimilation: The health of our digestive system, particularly the gut, influences the assimilation and absorption of energy from the foods we consume. A healthy gut microbiome, supported by a diet rich in fiber, probiotics, and prebiotics, promotes optimal digestion, nutrient absorption, and the efficient assimilation of energy from food. Nurturing gut health through a diverse and balanced diet enhances the energy body's ability to extract and utilize vital life force energy.

8. Essential Nutrients for Energy: Proper nutrition provides the body with essential nutrients that are vital for energy production and the functioning of the energy body. B vitamins, found in whole grains, legumes, and leafy greens, play a crucial role in energy metabolism. Magnesium, abundant in nuts, seeds, and leafy greens, supports cellular energy

Supplements and herbs for energy medicine

In the realm of energy medicine, supplements and herbs serve as valuable tools for promoting vitality, balance, and overall well-being. These natural remedies offer a wide range of benefits that support the body's subtle energy systems and enhance our energetic vitality. By understanding the role of supplements and herbs in energy medicine, individuals can harness their potential to optimize their energetic health. Below we will explore the relationship between supplements, herbs, and energy medicine, uncovering the benefits, considerations, and practical applications of these natural allies for supporting our energy systems.

2. Supplements and Energetic Balance: Supplements are concentrated sources of nutrients that support the body's overall health and energy balance. In energy medicine, certain supplements can specifically target the

subtle energy systems, nourishing and optimizing their function. Supplements such as vitamins, minerals, amino acids, and fatty acids provide the building blocks necessary for energy production, cellular function, and the well-being of our energy systems.

3. Adaptogens: Adaptogens are herbs and substances that help the body adapt to physical, mental, and emotional stressors, promoting resilience and balance. These herbs, such as ashwagandha, rhodiola, and ginseng, have been used for centuries in traditional medicine systems. Adaptogens support the body's stress response, enhance energy levels, and promote overall vitality. They are known for their ability to modulate the body's energy systems, promoting homeostasis and adaptability.

4. Herbal Tonics: Herbal tonics are preparations made from specific herbs or combinations of herbs that provide targeted support for the body's systems, including the energy body. These tonics often consist of herbs such as astragalus, schisandra, and licorice, which have adaptogenic, immune-supporting, and energizing properties. Herbal tonics nourish and strengthen the energy systems, supporting their optimal functioning and vitality.

5. Ayurvedic Rasayanas: Rasayanas are rejuvenating substances in Ayurvedic medicine that promote vitality, longevity, and the overall well-being of the body and energy systems. These substances can include herbs, minerals, and specialized formulations. Ayurvedic rasayanas, such as triphala, ashwagandha, and shilajit, help balance the energy systems, enhance vitality, and support the body's natural healing processes.

6. Essential Fatty Acids: Essential fatty acids, such as omega-3 and omega-6 fatty acids, play a vital role in energy production, brain function, and the health of the nervous system. These healthy fats are found in sources like fish oil, flaxseed oil, chia seeds, and walnuts. Essential fatty acids support

the integrity of the energy systems, enhance cellular communication, and promote overall energetic balance.

7. Antioxidants: Antioxidants are substances that help protect the body's cells and energy systems from oxidative stress and free radical damage. They neutralize harmful molecules that can disrupt the flow of energy and lead to imbalances within the energy body. Antioxidant-rich supplements, such as vitamin C, vitamin E, and resveratrol, support the overall health and vitality of the energy systems.

8. Flower Essences: Flower essences are energetic preparations made from the blossoms of specific flowers. These essences capture the energetic imprint of the flower and can be used to support emotional well-being and balance within the energy body. Flower essences, like Bach flower remedies, are commonly used in energy medicine to address emotional imbalances, promote positive energetic states, and support overall energetic harmony.

9. Herbal Teas: Herbal teas are an ancient and soothing way to support the energy systems. Different herbs have varying energetic

Chapter Thirteen

Energy Medicine and Sleep

Sleep is a fundamental aspect of our well-being, influencing our physical, mental, and emotional health. It is during sleep that our bodies repair, restore, and recharge, preparing us for the demands of the day ahead. In the realm of energy medicine, sleep is recognized as a vital time for the body's subtle energy systems to rejuvenate and rebalance. By understanding the connection between energy medicine and sleep, we can explore various techniques and practices that support restful nights and enhance our overall energetic vitality. Below we will delve into the relationship between energy medicine and sleep, uncovering the benefits, considerations, and practical strategies for nurturing our sleep and energetic well-being.

2. Sleep and Energetic Balance: Energy medicine acknowledges that quality sleep is essential for maintaining energetic balance within the body. During sleep, the body's energy systems undergo restoration and harmonization. Adequate sleep supports the flow of energy, optimizes cellular function, and promotes overall energetic vitality. Conversely, insufficient or disrupted sleep can lead to imbalances in the body's energy systems and impact overall well-being.

3. Creating a Sleep-Friendly Environment: Energy medicine emphasizes the importance of creating a sleep-friendly environment that promotes relaxation and restfulness. Factors such as comfortable bedding, a cool and dark room, and a quiet and serene ambiance can support the body's ability to enter a deep and rejuvenating sleep state. Creating a nurturing

sleep environment enhances the body's energetic receptivity to restorative energies.

4. Energetic Clearing and Pre-Sleep Rituals: Energetic clearing practices, such as smudging with sage or using essential oils, can help cleanse and harmonize the energy of the sleep environment. Pre-sleep rituals, such as meditation, deep breathing exercises, or gentle stretches, can calm the mind, release tension, and prepare the body for rest. These practices facilitate the transition from the active state of wakefulness to the receptive state of sleep.

5. Energetic Support with Crystals: Crystals are often used in energy medicine to support various aspects of well-being, including sleep. Certain crystals, such as amethyst, selenite, and moonstone, are known for their calming and soothing energies. Placing these crystals near the bed or under the pillow can help create a peaceful and energetically supportive sleep environment.

6. Energy Balancing Techniques: Energy medicine techniques, such as Reiki, Healing Touch, or Quantum Touch, can be applied to promote energetic balance and relaxation before sleep. These modalities work with the body's energy systems, promoting the release of tension, clearing energetic blockages, and restoring the flow of vital life force energy. By receiving energy balancing sessions or practicing self-healing techniques, individuals can enhance their energetic state and improve the quality of their sleep.

7. Mindfulness and Relaxation Techniques: Mindfulness practices, such as meditation, mindfulness-based stress reduction, or progressive muscle relaxation, can be powerful tools for promoting restful sleep. These techniques cultivate present-moment awareness, reduce mental chatter, and induce a state of deep relaxation. By practicing mindfulness and relaxation

techniques before bed, individuals can calm the mind, release stress, and prepare the body for a rejuvenating sleep experience.

8. Herbal Remedies and Essential Oils: Herbal remedies and essential oils have long been used for their soothing and sedative properties. Herbs such as chamomile, lavender, and valerian root have calming effects on the nervous system and promote relaxation. Essential oils, when diffused or applied topically, can enhance the sleep environment and facilitate a restful state of mind and body. Using herbal remedies and essential oils in conjunction with energy medicine practices can create a synergistic effect, supporting restful

Sleep disturbances and energy imbalances

Sleep is a vital aspect of our overall well-being, influencing our physical, mental, and emotional health. However, many individuals experience sleep disturbances, such as insomnia, restless sleep, or nightmares, which can disrupt the restorative nature of sleep and affect their daily functioning. In the realm of energy medicine, sleep disturbances are seen as indicators of underlying energy imbalances within the body. By understanding the connection between sleep disturbances and energy imbalances, we can explore how energy medicine techniques and practices can restore harmony, promote restful sleep, and enhance our overall energetic well-being. Below we will delve into the relationship between sleep disturbances and energy imbalances, uncovering the benefits, considerations, and practical strategies for restoring balance through energy medicine.

2. Sleep Disturbances as Energy Imbalances: Energy medicine recognizes that sleep disturbances can be manifestations of underlying energy imbalances within the body's subtle energy systems. Imbalances in the flow, distribution, or quality of energy can disrupt the body's ability to enter

and maintain a restful sleep state. Identifying and addressing these energy imbalances can help restore harmony and promote restorative sleep.

3. Blocked or Stagnant Energy: Blocked or stagnant energy within the body can contribute to sleep disturbances. Energy blockages can occur due to physical or emotional stress, trauma, or chronic tension. These blockages disrupt the flow of vital life force energy, leading to restlessness, difficulty falling asleep, or waking up feeling unrefreshed. Energy medicine techniques, such as acupuncture, acupressure, or Reiki, can help release these blockages, allowing energy to flow freely and promoting restful sleep.

4. Energetic Imbalances in Specific Energy Centers: Energy medicine recognizes that energy imbalances in specific energy centers or chakras can influence sleep patterns. For example, imbalances in the root chakra, which is associated with stability and security, can contribute to feelings of anxiety or restlessness at night. Similarly, imbalances in the third eye chakra, related to intuition and perception, can result in vivid dreams or nightmares. Balancing and harmonizing these energy centers through energy medicine practices can help alleviate sleep disturbances associated with specific chakra imbalances.

5. Stress and Energetic Overload: Chronic stress and energetic overload can disrupt the body's ability to relax and enter a restful sleep state. Stress triggers the release of stress hormones, which can keep the body in a heightened state of arousal, making it difficult to unwind and fall asleep. Energy medicine techniques, such as breathing exercises, meditation, or energy clearing practices, can help release stress and restore energetic balance, promoting a state of relaxation conducive to restful sleep.

6. Emotional Imbalances and Sleep: Emotions play a significant role in our sleep patterns. Negative emotions, such as anxiety, fear, or sadness, can contribute to sleep disturbances. Energy medicine approaches, like

Emotional Freedom Techniques (EFT) or energy psychology, help address and release emotional imbalances, promoting emotional well-being and improving sleep quality. By working with the body's energy systems, these techniques can help alleviate emotional imbalances that interfere with sleep.

7. Energetic Hygiene and Sleep Rituals: Energetic hygiene practices and sleep rituals can create a conducive environment for restful sleep. Energetic hygiene involves practices such as smudging, using essential oils, or energy clearing techniques to cleanse the sleep environment of stagnant or negative energy. Sleep rituals, like relaxation exercises, journaling, or gratitude practices, help calm the mind, release tension, and prepare the body for sleep. Engaging in these rituals fosters a sense of relaxation and supports the body's transition into a restful sleep state.

Supporting the Energy

Techniques for improving sleep quality

A good night's sleep is essential for our overall well-being and vitality. However, many individuals struggle with sleep-related issues that affect the quality and restorative nature of their rest. In the realm of energy medicine, various techniques can be employed to enhance sleep quality and promote a deeper and more rejuvenating slumber. By understanding the connection between energy medicine and sleep, we can explore practical strategies and approaches that foster restful nights and support our energetic well-being. Below we will delve into techniques for improving sleep quality through energy medicine, shedding light on their benefits, considerations, and practical applications.

2. Establishing a Sleep Routine: Consistency and routine are crucial for optimizing sleep quality. Energy medicine emphasizes the importance of

establishing a regular sleep routine by going to bed and waking up at the same time every day, including weekends. A consistent sleep schedule helps regulate the body's internal clock, aligning it with natural circadian rhythms and promoting better sleep quality.

3. Creating a Sleep-Friendly Environment: The sleep environment plays a significant role in promoting restful sleep. Energy medicine suggests creating a sleep-friendly environment that is cool, dark, and quiet. Consider using blackout curtains or an eye mask to block out light, earplugs or white noise machines to minimize noise disruptions, and a comfortable mattress and pillows that support proper alignment and comfort. By optimizing the sleep environment, we can create a sanctuary that promotes relaxation and enhances sleep quality.

4. Limiting Electronic Device Use: Electronic devices emit blue light that can disrupt the body's natural sleep-wake cycle by suppressing the production of melatonin, a hormone that regulates sleep. Energy medicine advises limiting exposure to electronic devices, such as smartphones, tablets, and computers, especially in the hours leading up to bedtime. Instead, engaging in calming activities like reading a book or practicing relaxation techniques can help prepare the mind and body for sleep.

5. Breathwork and Relaxation Techniques: Energy medicine recognizes the power of breathwork and relaxation techniques in promoting deep relaxation and preparing the body for sleep. Techniques such as diaphragmatic breathing, progressive muscle relaxation, or guided imagery can help calm the nervous system, release tension, and induce a state of deep relaxation. These practices support the body's natural transition into the sleep state.

6. Energetic Clearing and Grounding: Energetic clearing and grounding practices can help release accumulated stress and tension from the day,

allowing the body to relax and facilitate better sleep. Energy medicine techniques, such as smudging with sage, using essential oils, or energy clearing exercises, help cleanse the energy field, release energetic blockages, and promote a sense of calm and balance. Grounding techniques, such as walking barefoot on grass or practicing grounding visualizations, can also help establish a connection with the earth's energy, promoting relaxation and facilitating deeper sleep.

7. Meditation and Mindfulness: Meditation and mindfulness practices are valuable tools for quieting the mind, reducing mental chatter, and cultivating a state of inner calm. Energy medicine encourages incorporating meditation or mindfulness into bedtime routines to help calm racing thoughts, promote relaxation, and facilitate a smooth transition into sleep. Guided meditation apps or gentle body scan techniques can be particularly useful in this regard.

8. Energy Balancing Techniques: Energy medicine techniques, such as Reiki, Healing Touch, or acupuncture, can help balance the body's energy systems, release stagnant energy, and promote the free flow of vital life force energy. These techniques help address energetic imbalances that may contribute to sleep disturbances, supporting overall well-being and improving sleep quality. By receiving energy balancing sessions or practicing self-healing techniques, individuals can optimize their energetic state and enhance the quality of their sleep.

Herbal Teas and

The role of energy medicine in treating sleep disorders

Sleep disorders can significantly impact an individual's overall well-being, affecting their physical health, cognitive function, and emotional stability. In recent years, energy medicine has emerged as a promising approach for treating sleep disorders by addressing the underlying energetic imbalances that contribute to disrupted sleep patterns. Energy medicine recognizes the interconnectedness of the body, mind, and energy systems, offering a holistic framework for understanding and treating sleep disturbances. Below we will explore the role of energy medicine in treating sleep disorders, examining its benefits, considerations, and practical applications in promoting healthy sleep patterns.

2. Understanding Energetic Imbalances in Sleep Disorders: Energy medicine views sleep disorders as manifestations of underlying energetic imbalances within the body's subtle energy systems. These imbalances can arise from factors such as stress, trauma, emotional blockages, or disruptions in the flow of vital life force energy. By identifying and addressing these imbalances, energy medicine aims to restore harmony within the energy systems and promote healthy sleep patterns.

3. Energy Assessment and Diagnosis: Energy medicine practitioners utilize various assessment techniques, such as visual observation, palpation, or energetic scanning, to identify energetic imbalances that may contribute to sleep disorders. These assessments help determine the state of the body's energy systems, identify blockages or disturbances, and inform personalized treatment plans. By understanding the unique energetic makeup of each individual, energy medicine practitioners can tailor interventions to address specific sleep-related issues.

Energy-Based Techniques for Sleep Disorders: Energy medicine offers a range of techniques and modalities that can be effective in treating sleep disorders. These techniques focus on rebalancing the body's energy systems, releasing energetic blockages, and promoting the free flow of vital life force energy. Some commonly used energy-based techniques include:

4. Reiki: Reiki is a Japanese technique that involves the gentle laying of hands on specific areas of the body to channel healing energy. It aims to balance the body's energy, promote relaxation, and support overall well-being. Reiki can be beneficial in addressing the energetic imbalances underlying sleep disorders and promoting a state of deep relaxation conducive to restful sleep.

5. Acupuncture: Acupuncture is an ancient Chinese practice that involves the insertion of thin needles into specific points along the body's meridian pathways. By stimulating these points, acupuncture aims to restore the balance and flow of energy within the body. Acupuncture has shown promise in treating sleep disorders, such as insomnia or sleep apnea, by addressing the underlying energetic imbalances.

6. Energy Psychology: Energy psychology approaches, such as Emotional Freedom Techniques (EFT) or Thought Field Therapy (TFT), combine energy-based interventions with psychological principles. These techniques involve tapping on specific acupressure points while focusing on sleep-related issues or emotional disturbances. Energy psychology can help release emotional blockages and promote relaxation, leading to improved sleep quality.

7. Chakra Balancing: Energy medicine recognizes the role of the chakra system in regulating energy flow within the body. The chakras are energy centers located along the central channel of the body, and each chakra is associated with specific physical, emotional, and energetic functions. Imbalances in the chakras can impact sleep patterns. Techniques such as chakra balancing, using crystals, sound therapy, or visualization, can help restore the flow of energy through the chakras, promoting overall energetic balance and improving sleep quality.

8. Mind-Body Practices: Energy medicine recognizes the profound influence of the mind-body connection on sleep patterns. Techniques such as meditation, guided imagery, or breathwork help calm the mind, reduce stress, and promote a state of deep relaxation. These practices support the body's natural transition into sleep, helping to alleviate sleep disorders by addressing the underlying energetic im

Chapter Fourteen

Energy Medicine for Children and Teens

Energy medicine is a holistic approach that recognizes the interconnectedness of the body, mind, and energy systems. While traditionally associated with adults, energy medicine is also gaining recognition as a valuable tool for promoting the health and well-being of children and teenagers. By addressing the subtle energy systems, energy medicine offers a safe and effective means to support healthy development, address emotional and physical challenges, and enhance overall well-being in the younger population. Below we will explore the role of energy medicine for children and teens, examining its benefits, considerations, and practical applications in nurturing their well-being.

2. Energetic Awareness and Education: Energy medicine introduces children and teens to the concept of subtle energy and its impact on their overall health and well-being. Through age-appropriate education, children and teens can develop a deeper understanding of their energetic bodies, learn to recognize their own energy, and explore techniques for self-care and emotional regulation. Energetic awareness empowers young individuals to take an active role in nurturing their own well-being.

3. Emotional Regulation and Stress Management: Children and teens often face emotional challenges, such as stress, anxiety, or anger. Energy medicine offers effective tools for emotional regulation and stress management. Techniques such as EFT (Emotional Freedom Techniques), which involve tapping on specific acupressure points, or breathing exercises, help

children and teens release emotional blockages, reduce stress levels, and cultivate emotional resilience. These practices provide valuable coping mechanisms and support healthy emotional development.

4. Balancing the Energy Systems: Energy imbalances can affect children and teens, impacting their physical, emotional, and mental well-being. Energy medicine techniques, such as Reiki, Healing Touch, or chakra balancing, help restore harmony and balance within the energy systems. These modalities promote the free flow of vital life force energy, enhance overall vitality, and support the body's natural healing mechanisms. Balancing the energy systems can address a wide range of issues, including sleep disturbances, pain, and emotional challenges.

5. Support for Neurodevelopmental Conditions: Energy medicine shows promise in supporting children and teens with neurodevelopmental conditions, such as autism spectrum disorder (ASD) or attention deficit hyperactivity disorder (ADHD). Energy-based interventions, combined with other therapeutic approaches, can help reduce sensory sensitivities, promote relaxation, and support improved focus and attention. These techniques offer a gentle and non-invasive alternative or complement to traditional therapies.

6. Enhancing Mind-Body Connection: Energy medicine emphasizes the mind-body connection, recognizing that mental and emotional well-being are closely intertwined with physical health. Mind-body practices, such as meditation, visualization, or guided imagery, help children and teens develop a deeper connection with their bodies, cultivate self-awareness, and promote overall well-being. These practices foster a sense of inner calm, self-acceptance, and positive self-image.

7. Promoting Healthy Sleep Patterns: Sleep is crucial for the growth and development of children and teens. Energy medicine techniques can help

address sleep disturbances and promote healthy sleep patterns. Energetic clearing practices, bedtime rituals, or relaxation techniques can create a calming sleep environment, release accumulated stress, and support a restful sleep state. By addressing the underlying energy imbalances and establishing healthy sleep habits, energy medicine contributes to overall well-being and cognitive function.

8. Energetic Protection and Grounding: Children and teens may encounter challenging or overwhelming energetic environments, such as crowded places or school settings. Energy medicine teaches techniques for energetic protection and grounding. Visualization exercises, the use of protective crystals, or simple grounding practices help children and teens establish energetic boundaries, enhance their resilience, and maintain a sense of stability and balance in their daily lives.

Supporting Self-Expression and

Supporting children's energy systems

Children are naturally vibrant, energetic beings who possess a unique and delicate energy system. Just as adults benefit from the principles and practices of energy medicine, children can also benefit from its gentle yet powerful approach. Energy medicine offers a holistic framework for supporting children's energy systems, promoting balance, emotional well-being, and overall vitality. By understanding the role of energy medicine in supporting children's energy systems, we can explore effective strategies and practices that contribute to their optimal growth and development. Below we will delve into the importance of supporting children's energy systems through energy medicine, highlighting its benefits, considerations, and practical applications.

2. Energetic Awareness and Education: Energy medicine encourages children to develop an understanding of their own energy systems from an early age. By introducing simple concepts and terminology, children can learn about the flow of energy in their bodies and its connection to their overall well-being. Energetic education helps children develop a sense of self-awareness and empowers them to take an active role in nurturing their own energy.

3. Emotional Regulation and Stress Management: Children often experience a wide range of emotions and face various stressors in their daily lives. Energy medicine provides effective tools for emotional regulation and stress management. Techniques such as breathing exercises, visualization, or tapping can help children release emotional tension, reduce stress levels, and cultivate emotional resilience. These practices empower children to navigate their emotions and establish healthy coping mechanisms.

4. Balancing the Energy Centers: Energy medicine recognizes the presence of energy centers, often referred to as chakras, within the body. These centers play a crucial role in the flow and distribution of energy. Supporting children's energy systems involves harmonizing and balancing these energy centers. Techniques such as chakra balancing, crystal therapy, or gentle energy touch can help clear blockages, restore balance, and enhance overall energy flow in children.

5. Support for Sensory Sensitivities: Many children have heightened sensory sensitivities, which can impact their overall well-being and daily functioning. Energy medicine techniques, such as energy clearing or shielding, can help children manage sensory overload and protect their energy fields. Grounding exercises, visualization, or the use of calming essential oils can also support children in navigating sensory sensitivities and finding balance in their energetic experiences.

6. Enhancing Creativity and Imagination: Energy medicine recognizes the power of creativity and imagination in supporting children's energy systems. Encouraging creative expression, such as drawing, painting, storytelling, or engaging in imaginative play, helps children tap into their innate energetic potential. These activities allow energy to flow freely, promote self-expression, and stimulate the development of their energetic capacities.

7. Promoting Healthy Boundaries: Supporting children's energy systems involves teaching them about personal boundaries and energetic hygiene. Energy medicine emphasizes the importance of establishing healthy boundaries, both physical and energetic, to protect their well-being. Teaching children techniques for energetic protection, such as visualization exercises or setting intentions, empowers them to maintain healthy boundaries in various environments and interactions.

8. Nurturing Connection with Nature: Nature serves as a powerful source of energy and nourishment for children's energy systems. Spending time outdoors, engaging in nature walks, gardening, or other nature-based activities helps children connect with the Earth's natural energy. These experiences enhance their grounding, promote a sense of interconnectedness, and support the balanced development of their energy systems.

9. Parental and Caregiver Involvement: Supporting children's energy systems requires the involvement of parents and caregivers. They play a vital role in creating an energetically supportive environment at home. Parents can engage in energy-clearing practices, create calming and nurturing spaces, and model healthy energetic boundaries. Additionally, caregivers can learn basic energy medicine techniques

Energy medicine techniques for teens

The teenage years are a time of immense growth, self-discovery, and emotional development. As teenagers navigate the challenges and transitions of adolescence, energy medicine offers valuable techniques to support their well-being and enhance their self-care practices. By incorporating energy medicine into their daily routines, teens can cultivate a deeper understanding of their own energy systems, manage stress, and foster emotional resilience. Below we will explore a range of energy medicine techniques specifically tailored to teens, highlighting their benefits, considerations, and practical applications.

2. Breathwork and Mindful Awareness: Breathwork is a powerful tool for managing stress, enhancing focus, and promoting emotional well-being. Techniques such as deep diaphragmatic breathing, alternate nostril breathing, or box breathing help teens regulate their nervous system, reduce anxiety, and increase their overall energetic balance. Mindful awareness of the breath allows teens to connect with their inner state, promoting a sense of calm and centeredness.

3. Emotional Freedom Techniques (EFT): EFT, also known as tapping, is a gentle yet effective energy psychology technique. By tapping on specific acupressure points while focusing on negative emotions or challenging experiences, teens can release emotional blockages, reduce anxiety, and promote emotional well-being. EFT empowers teens to process and manage their emotions, supporting their mental and energetic equilibrium.

4. Chakra Balancing: Energy medicine recognizes the presence of energy centers, or chakras, within the body. Each chakra is associated with specific qualities and functions. Teens can benefit from chakra balancing practices to restore harmony and enhance their energy flow. Simple techniques, such as visualization, meditation, or working with crystals, can help teens align and balance their chakras, fostering emotional and energetic well-being.

5. Grounding and Earthing: Grounding techniques help teens connect with the Earth's energy, promoting stability, and emotional balance. Walking barefoot on grass or sand, spending time in nature, or visualizing roots extending from their feet into the Earth are effective grounding practices. Grounding allows teens to release excess energy, reduce feelings of overwhelm, and cultivate a sense of stability and security.

6. Visualization and Guided Imagery: Visualization is a powerful tool for teens to tap into their imaginative capacities and support their energetic well-being. Guided imagery practices, whether led by a teacher or accessed through audio recordings, help teens relax, reduce stress, and enhance their self-awareness. Visualization allows teens to explore their inner world, cultivate positive self-image, and manifest their goals and aspirations.

7. Energy Clearing and Smudging: Teens can benefit from energy clearing techniques to release accumulated stress, negative energy, or emotional residue. Smudging with sage or using other energy-clearing tools, such as sound or essential oils, helps cleanse their personal energy field and create a sense of energetic renewal. Energy clearing practices support emotional well-being and create a positive energetic environment for teens.

8. Self-Healing Practices: Teens can learn and practice self-healing techniques to nurture their emotional well-being. Simple practices such as placing hands on specific areas of the body, using affirmations or positive self-talk, and applying gentle touch promote self-awareness, self-compassion, and energetic balance. Encouraging teens to explore self-healing practices empowers them to take an active role in their own well-being.

9. Mindfulness Meditation: Mindfulness meditation teaches teens to be present in the moment, cultivate non-judgmental awareness, and reduce stress. Mindfulness practices help teens develop a deeper connection with their own experiences, emotions, and thoughts, enhancing self-regulation

and resilience. By practicing mindfulness meditation, teens can improve focus, reduce anxiety, and foster a sense of inner

Addressing common childhood and adolescent issues with energy medicine

Childhood and adolescence are transformative periods filled with growth, exploration, and unique challenges. Energy medicine offers a holistic approach to address common issues that children and adolescents may encounter during these formative years. By working with the subtle energy systems of the body, energy medicine techniques provide gentle and effective solutions for promoting well-being, emotional balance, and resilience. Below we will explore how energy medicine can address common childhood and adolescent issues, highlighting its benefits, considerations, and practical applications.

2. Anxiety and Stress Reduction: Anxiety and stress are prevalent issues among children and adolescents. Energy medicine techniques, such as Emotional Freedom Techniques (EFT), breathing exercises, or visualization, can help reduce anxiety levels and promote emotional balance. These practices empower children and teens to manage stress, regulate their nervous system, and cultivate emotional resilience.

3. Emotional Regulation and Self-Expression: Emotional challenges are common during childhood and adolescence. Energy medicine provides tools for emotional regulation and self-expression. Techniques like EFT, chakra balancing, or journaling allow children and teens to process emotions, release emotional blockages, and develop healthy coping mechanisms. These practices foster self-awareness, self-acceptance, and emotional well-being.

4. ADHD and Focus Enhancement: Attention deficit hyperactivity disorder (ADHD) can impact a child's ability to concentrate and stay focused. Energy medicine techniques, such as mindfulness meditation, grounding exercises, or acupressure, can support children with ADHD by promoting a sense of calm, enhancing focus, and improving attention span. These practices help regulate energy flow and support cognitive function.

5. Behavioral Issues and Anger Management: Some children and adolescents struggle with behavioral issues or difficulty managing anger. Energy medicine techniques offer effective strategies for anger management and behavior regulation. EFT, breathing exercises, or energy grounding practices can help release anger, reduce emotional reactivity, and promote emotional self-regulation. These techniques support emotional balance and healthier interpersonal interactions.

6. Sleep Disturbances and Insomnia: Sleep disturbances can significantly impact a child's physical and emotional well-being. Energy medicine techniques can address underlying energy imbalances that contribute to sleep issues. Practices such as relaxation exercises, energy clearing rituals, or bedtime visualization can help children and teens relax, release tension, and promote restful sleep. By restoring energetic balance, these techniques support healthy sleep patterns.

7. Self-Esteem and Body Image: Self-esteem and body image issues can arise during childhood and adolescence. Energy medicine techniques foster self-acceptance and positive self-image. Chakra balancing, visualization exercises, or affirmations empower children and teens to cultivate self-worth, appreciate their unique qualities, and develop a healthy relationship with their bodies. These practices support a positive sense of self and overall well-being.

8. Social Anxiety and Peer Pressure: Social anxiety and peer pressure are common challenges for children and teens. Energy medicine techniques can help alleviate social anxiety by promoting self-confidence, reducing stress, and enhancing social-emotional skills. Practices like EFT, grounding exercises, or mindful breathing can support children and teens in navigating social situations with greater ease, assertiveness, and resilience.

9. Trauma and Emotional Healing: Children and adolescents may experience trauma, whether from a single event or ongoing stressors. Energy medicine provides effective tools for emotional healing and trauma release. Techniques like EFT, energy clearing, or Reiki can help release trapped emotions, restore energetic balance, and promote overall well-being. These practices support the healing process and empower children and teens to process their experiences in a safe and nurturing way.

10. Academic Performance and Concentration: Academic performance and concentration are important aspects of a child's development. Energy medicine techniques offer support for improved cognitive function and academic success

Chapter Fifteen

Energy Medicine for Aging and Longevity

Aging is a natural part of life, and with it comes a desire for vitality, well-being, and a fulfilling quality of life. Energy medicine offers a holistic approach to support aging individuals in maintaining their health, enhancing their vitality, and promoting longevity. By working with the body's subtle energy systems, energy medicine techniques address the energetic imbalances that can contribute to physical and emotional challenges commonly associated with aging. Below we will explore how energy medicine can be utilized to support aging and promote longevity, highlighting its benefits, considerations, and practical applications.

2. Understanding Energy Systems in Aging: Energy medicine recognizes that the human body is composed of intricate energy systems that play a vital role in our overall well-being. As we age, these energy systems may become imbalanced, leading to various physical and emotional issues. By understanding and working with these energy systems, energy medicine offers a means to restore balance, support optimal functioning, and enhance vitality in the aging process.

3. Promoting Physical Well-being: Energy medicine techniques can address physical challenges commonly experienced in aging. Practices such as Reiki, acupuncture, or therapeutic touch can help restore the flow of energy, alleviate pain, and support the body's natural healing mechanisms. By working with the body's energy systems, energy medicine offers a com-

plementary approach to conventional medical interventions, promoting physical well-being and enhancing the body's ability to heal itself.

4. Emotional and Mental Health Support: Aging is often accompanied by emotional and mental changes. Energy medicine provides tools for promoting emotional and mental well-being in the later years of life. Techniques such as Emotional Freedom Techniques (EFT), energy psychology, or meditation can help release emotional blockages, reduce anxiety or depression, and foster emotional resilience. These practices empower aging individuals to navigate life's transitions with a greater sense of emotional balance and well-being.

5. Enhancing Cognitive Function: Cognitive decline is a common concern associated with aging. Energy medicine techniques can support brain health and enhance cognitive function. Practices such as mindfulness meditation, visualization, or brainwave entrainment can help improve focus, concentration, and memory. These techniques promote neuroplasticity and support healthy brain aging, contributing to overall cognitive well-being.

6. Managing Chronic Illness and Pain: Chronic illness and pain can significantly impact the quality of life in aging individuals. Energy medicine offers alternative approaches to managing chronic conditions and alleviating pain. Techniques such as energy healing, acupuncture, or sound therapy can help reduce symptoms, support the body's self-healing mechanisms, and enhance overall well-being. By addressing the underlying energetic imbalances, energy medicine provides a holistic perspective on managing chronic conditions.

7. Promoting Vitality and Energy: Energy medicine focuses on restoring and enhancing the body's vital life force energy. Techniques such as chakra balancing, energy clearing, or breathwork can help revitalize the energy

systems, boost vitality, and promote a sense of rejuvenation. These practices contribute to overall energy and well-being, allowing aging individuals to maintain an active and fulfilling lifestyle.

8. Supporting Healthy Sleep Patterns: Sleep disturbances are common among older adults. Energy medicine techniques can address the underlying energetic imbalances that contribute to sleep issues. Practices such as energy clearing rituals, relaxation exercises, or bedtime visualization can promote relaxation, release tension, and support restful sleep. By restoring energetic balance, energy medicine contributes to healthy sleep patterns and enhances overall rejuvenation during sleep.

9. Nurturing Spirituality and Inner Connection: Aging often prompts contemplation of deeper existential questions and the search for meaning and purpose. Energy medicine acknowledges the spiritual dimension of life and offers techniques to nurture spirituality and inner connection. Practices such as meditation, contemplation, or energy-based rituals provide avenues for self-reflection

The impact of aging on the energy body

Aging is a natural process that brings about various physical, emotional, and energetic changes in the human body. Just as the physical body undergoes transformations with age, the energy body—comprised of subtle energy systems—also experiences shifts. Energy medicine recognizes the interconnectedness of the physical and energetic aspects of our being, and understanding the impact of aging on the energy body can provide insights into promoting well-being in the later stages of life. Below we will explore the impact of aging on the energy body, shedding light on the changes that occur and the implications for overall health and vitality.

2. Decline in Vital Life Force Energy: With age, there is a natural decline in the overall level of vital life force energy within the energy body. This decline can affect the functioning of the energy systems, leading to imbalances and decreased vitality. Energy medicine techniques aim to restore and replenish this vital energy, promoting well-being and supporting the body's natural healing processes.

3. Energetic Imbalances and Blockages: As we age, energetic imbalances and blockages may develop within the energy body. These imbalances can occur as a result of various factors, including emotional experiences, physical ailments, or energetic stagnation. Energy medicine techniques such as Reiki, acupuncture, or chakra balancing can help identify and address these imbalances, restoring the flow of energy and promoting overall energetic harmony.

4. Impact on Emotional Well-being: Aging can bring about emotional changes and challenges. The energy body plays a significant role in emotional well-being, and imbalances within the energy systems can contribute to emotional disturbances such as anxiety or depression. Energy medicine techniques such as Emotional Freedom Techniques (EFT), energy psychology, or meditation can help release emotional blockages, promote emotional resilience, and support healthy emotional well-being in the later stages of life.

5. Changes in Energy Centers: Energy centers, often referred to as chakras, are key components of the energy body. These centers play a vital role in the overall functioning of the energy system. As we age, changes can occur within the energy centers, affecting their balance and alignment. Energy medicine techniques like chakra balancing, visualization, or energy clearing can help restore and harmonize the energy centers, promoting a sense of balance and vitality.

6. Influence on Physical Health: The energy body and physical body are intimately connected. The energetic imbalances that arise with aging can impact physical health and well-being. Energy medicine techniques offer a holistic approach to address these imbalances, supporting physical health through practices such as energy healing, acupuncture, or therapeutic touch. By restoring energetic balance, energy medicine can contribute to overall physical vitality and promote optimal functioning of bodily systems.

7. Impact on Cognitive Function: Cognitive changes can accompany the aging process, including memory lapses or decreased mental clarity. The energy body plays a role in cognitive function, and energetic imbalances can contribute to cognitive decline. Energy medicine techniques such as mindfulness meditation, breathwork, or brainwave entrainment can support cognitive health, promoting focus, clarity, and mental acuity in the golden years.

8. Spiritual Reflection and Connection: Aging often prompts contemplation of deeper existential questions and the search for spiritual connection and meaning. The energy body serves as a conduit for spiritual experiences, and the aging process can provide opportunities for spiritual growth and introspection. Energy medicine practices such as meditation, contemplation, or energy-based rituals can facilitate spiritual reflection, fostering a sense of inner connection and deepening one's spiritual journey.

9. Importance of Energetic Self-Care: Understanding the impact of aging on the energy body emphasizes the importance of energetic self-care in the later stages of life. Engaging in regular energy medicine

Energy medicine techniques for graceful aging

Aging is a natural part of life, and how we navigate this process greatly impacts our overall well-being and quality of life. Energy medicine offers a holistic approach to support graceful aging by addressing the physical, emotional, and energetic aspects of our being. By utilizing specific energy medicine techniques, individuals can nurture vitality, promote well-being, and embrace the journey of aging with grace and resilience. Below we will explore a range of energy medicine techniques tailored for graceful aging, highlighting their benefits, considerations, and practical applications.

2. Chakra Balancing: Chakras are vital energy centers within the body that influence our physical, emotional, and spiritual well-being. As we age, imbalances can occur within these energy centers, affecting our overall vitality. Chakra balancing techniques, such as visualization, Reiki, or sound therapy, help restore harmony and optimal energy flow. By balancing the chakras, individuals can support their physical health, emotional balance, and spiritual connection.

3. Energy Clearing: Over time, energetic blockages and accumulated negative energy can hinder our vitality and well-being. Energy clearing techniques, such as smudging with sage, use of crystals, or sound healing, help release stagnant energy and promote a sense of renewal. Regular energy clearing rituals can contribute to the maintenance of a clear and vibrant energy field, supporting overall vitality and emotional well-being.

4. Breathwork and Pranayama: Breathwork practices are powerful tools for promoting vitality and relaxation. Techniques like deep diaphragmatic breathing or alternate nostril breathing can help calm the nervous system, reduce stress, and enhance energy flow throughout the body. Consistent practice of breathwork supports oxygenation, increases vitality, and cultivates a deep sense of relaxation and rejuvenation.

5. Mindfulness Meditation: Mindfulness meditation fosters present-moment awareness, cultivates a calm and focused mind, and supports emotional well-being. By incorporating mindfulness into daily life, individuals can reduce stress, enhance resilience, and promote a sense of inner peace. Regular mindfulness practice helps navigate the challenges and changes that come with aging, allowing for greater clarity and acceptance.

6. Emotional Freedom Techniques (EFT): Emotional well-being is a key aspect of graceful aging. EFT, also known as tapping, is a technique that combines acupressure and psychological processes to release emotional blockages and promote emotional balance. By gently tapping on specific meridian points while focusing on an emotional issue, individuals can alleviate emotional distress, reduce anxiety, and enhance emotional resilience.

7. Energy Healing: Energy healing modalities, such as Reiki, therapeutic touch, or Quantum Touch, facilitate the flow of energy, supporting the body's natural healing mechanisms. These practices help address energetic imbalances, reduce pain, and promote overall well-being. Energy healing sessions can be particularly beneficial for individuals experiencing physical discomfort or undergoing medical treatments.

8. Gentle Movement and Exercise: Engaging in gentle movement and exercise is crucial for maintaining physical health and vitality. Energy medicine approaches, such as Tai Chi, Qigong, or Yoga, combine mindful movement with breath awareness, promoting flexibility, balance, and energy flow. These practices support joint mobility, improve posture, and enhance overall physical vitality.

9. Sound Therapy: Sound has a profound effect on our energy field and well-being. Sound therapy techniques, such as singing bowls, tuning forks, or sound baths, can help restore energetic balance and promote relaxation. The vibrational frequencies produced by these instruments resonate with

the energy centers, releasing tension, promoting a sense of harmony, and supporting overall well-being.

10. Engaging with Nature: Connecting with nature is essential for graceful aging. Spending time outdoors, walking barefoot on the Earth, or

Longevity practices and energy medicine

Longevity, the desire for a long and fulfilling life, has been a pursuit of humanity throughout history. While genetics and lifestyle factors play a role in the aging process, energy medicine offers additional tools to support health, vitality, and longevity. By working with the body's subtle energy systems, individuals can engage in practices that promote longevity and enhance overall well-being. Below we will explore a range of longevity practices in relation to energy medicine, highlighting their benefits, considerations, and practical applications.

2. Mind-Body Connection: The mind-body connection is a key component of longevity practices. Energy medicine recognizes that the state of our mind and emotions influences our physical health. Practices such as meditation, visualization, and affirmations promote a positive mindset, reduce stress, and support overall well-being. By fostering a harmonious mind-body connection, individuals can enhance their vitality and longevity.

3. Nutritional Support: Proper nutrition is essential for longevity and energy maintenance. Energy medicine emphasizes the importance of consuming nutrient-rich foods that support the body's energy systems. Fresh fruits and vegetables, whole grains, lean proteins, and healthy fats provide the necessary building blocks for optimal energy flow and cellular health. Individualized dietary recommendations based on energy assessments can further enhance nutritional support.

4. Detoxification: Detoxification practices are integral to energy medicine and longevity. Toxins accumulated in the body can disrupt energy flow and contribute to premature aging. Techniques such as fasting, juicing, herbal remedies, or energy clearing rituals help remove toxins and promote the body's natural detoxification processes. By reducing the toxic burden, individuals support their energy systems and overall well-being.

5. Stress Reduction: Chronic stress is a major contributor to premature aging and disease. Energy medicine techniques such as meditation, deep breathing, and stress reduction exercises help individuals manage stress levels and promote relaxation. By reducing stress, individuals can optimize their energy flow, support their immune system, and enhance their longevity.

6. Movement and Exercise: Physical activity is crucial for maintaining vitality and longevity. Energy medicine encourages individuals to engage in regular exercise that supports the body's energy systems. Practices such as Tai Chi, Qigong, Yoga, or other gentle movement modalities promote flexibility, balance, and energy flow. By incorporating mindful movement into daily routines, individuals can enhance their vitality and support overall well-being.

7. Sleep and Restorative Practices: Quality sleep is essential for rejuvenation and longevity. Energy medicine highlights the importance of restorative practices such as maintaining a consistent sleep schedule, creating a relaxing sleep environment, and engaging in relaxation techniques before bed. Adequate restful sleep allows the body's energy systems to recharge, supports cellular repair, and enhances overall vitality.

8. Energetic Self-Care: Energetic self-care is a foundational aspect of energy medicine and longevity practices. Techniques such as energy clearing rituals, self-massage, or working with crystals promote the balance and

flow of energy. By incorporating regular energetic self-care practices into daily routines, individuals can support their energy systems, reduce energetic imbalances, and enhance their overall well-being.

9. Social Connections and Emotional Support: Meaningful social connections and emotional well-being contribute to longevity. Energy medicine recognizes the importance of healthy relationships and emotional balance. Practices such as EFT (Emotional Freedom Techniques), energy psychology, or energy balancing exercises support emotional well-being, foster positive relationships, and enhance overall vitality.

10. Mindful Aging and Wisdom Cultivation: Mindful aging is a key component of longevity practices. Embracing the wisdom that comes with age and cultivating gratitude, acceptance, and self-reflection contribute to a fulfilling and meaningful life. Energy medicine techniques, such as journaling, meditation, or guided imagery,

Chapter Sixteen

Energy Medicine for Relationships

Relationships are an integral part of our human experience, influencing our well-being, happiness, and personal growth. Energy medicine recognizes that relationships are not solely based on external interactions but are also deeply influenced by the subtle energies that flow between individuals. By understanding and working with these energetic dynamics, we can cultivate healthier and more harmonious relationships. Below we will explore how energy medicine can enhance relationships, promote connection, and nurture emotional well-being, highlighting its benefits, considerations, and practical applications.

2. Energetic Awareness: Energy medicine emphasizes the importance of developing energetic awareness in relationships. Each individual has their own unique energetic signature, which interacts and intertwines with others. By cultivating awareness of our own energy and the energy of others, we can navigate relationships with greater sensitivity, empathy, and understanding.

3. Clearing and Balancing: Energetic imbalances can affect the dynamics of relationships. Energy medicine techniques such as Reiki, energy clearing rituals, or breathwork can help clear and balance the energy within ourselves and our relationships. These practices support the release of stagnant or negative energy, fostering a more harmonious energetic exchange between individuals.

4. Communication and Empathy: Effective communication is essential for healthy relationships. Energy medicine techniques can enhance communication skills by promoting empathy, active listening, and intuitive understanding. Practices such as EFT (Emotional Freedom Techniques), energy grounding exercises, or mindfulness meditation can cultivate emotional awareness and promote deeper connections within relationships.

5. Healing Relationship Trauma: Past traumas or unresolved emotional wounds can impact current relationships. Energy medicine provides tools to address and heal relationship trauma, whether it stems from childhood experiences, previous partnerships, or ancestral patterns. Techniques such as energy healing, inner child work, or guided visualization can help release energetic imprints and promote healing within relationship dynamics.

6. Boundaries and Energetic Protection: Establishing healthy boundaries and energetic protection is crucial in maintaining balanced relationships. Energy medicine practices such as aura protection techniques, cord-cutting exercises, or visualization can support individuals in setting and maintaining boundaries, while also fostering a sense of energetic integrity within relationships. This allows for authentic connection while respecting individual needs and well-being.

7. Relationship Cord Clearing: Energetic cords can form between individuals, representing the energetic connections and attachments we have with others. While some cords may be positive and nurturing, others can be draining or limiting. Energy medicine techniques like cord cutting or energy clearing rituals can help release unhealthy cords, promoting freedom, autonomy, and healthier energetic dynamics within relationships.

8. Enhancing Intimacy and Connection: Energy medicine offers practices to deepen intimacy and connection within relationships. Techniques such as couples' energy healing sessions, partner meditations, or tantric prac-

tices promote energetic attunement, heart-centered communication, and a sense of oneness. These practices foster a deeper sense of love, trust, and intimacy between partners.

9. Supporting Emotional Resilience: Emotional well-being is vital for healthy relationships. Energy medicine techniques, including EFT, chakra balancing, or energy grounding exercises, can support emotional resilience and regulation within relationships. By addressing emotional imbalances, individuals can cultivate emotional awareness, respond to challenges with greater clarity, and maintain healthier emotional boundaries.

10. Cultivating Positive Relationship Patterns: Energy medicine empowers individuals to consciously create positive relationship patterns. Through visualization, affirmation, and energy-clearing techniques, individuals can release negative relationship patterns and cultivate new energetic templates for healthy and fulfilling relationships. This promotes a positive energetic resonance and attracts relationships that are aligned with one's highest well-being.

11. Relationship Rituals and Sacred Space: Creating sacred space and engaging in relationship rituals can deepen connection and strengthen the energetic bond between individuals. Energy medicine practices such as shared meditation,

The role of energy medicine in maintaining healthy relationships

Relationships are at the core of our human experience, shaping our lives, and influencing our overall well-being. Maintaining healthy and fulfilling relationships requires attention not only to our actions and emotions but also to the energetic dynamics that underlie these connections. Energy medicine offers valuable insights and practices to support the maintenance of healthy relationships by working with the subtle energies that flow between individuals. Below we will explore the role of energy medicine in fostering healthy relationships, promoting connection, and nurturing emotional well-being, highlighting its benefits, considerations, and practical applications.

2. Energetic Awareness: Energy medicine emphasizes the importance of cultivating energetic awareness in relationships. It recognizes that each individual carries a unique energetic signature, and these energies interact and intertwine when in relationship with others. By developing awareness of our own energy and the energy of others, we can navigate relationships with greater sensitivity, empathy, and understanding.

3. Balancing and Harmonizing Energies: Energetic imbalances can disrupt relationship dynamics. Energy medicine techniques, such as Reiki, chakra balancing, or energy clearing rituals, can help restore harmony and balance within ourselves and our relationships. By addressing energetic imbalances, we create a more harmonious energetic exchange, fostering healthier and more fulfilling connections.

4. Communication and Empathy: Effective communication is vital for maintaining healthy relationships. Energy medicine techniques can enhance communication skills by promoting empathy, active listening, and intuitive understanding. Practices such as heart-centered communication, energy grounding exercises, or mindfulness meditation foster emotional awareness, deepening connections within relationships.

5. Healing Relationship Wounds: Past traumas or unresolved emotional wounds can impact current relationships. Energy medicine provides tools to address and heal relationship wounds, whether they stem from childhood experiences, past partnerships, or ancestral patterns. Techniques such as energy healing, inner child work, or guided visualization can help

release energetic imprints and promote healing within relationship dynamics.

6. Establishing Boundaries and Energetic Protection: Setting and maintaining healthy boundaries is crucial for maintaining balanced relationships. Energy medicine practices, such as aura protection techniques, cord-cutting exercises, or visualization, support individuals in establishing boundaries and fostering a sense of energetic integrity within relationships. This allows for authentic connection while respecting individual needs and well-being.

7. Clearing Energetic Attachments: Energetic attachments, such as cords or energetic imprints, can form between individuals, impacting relationship dynamics. Energy medicine techniques, like cord cutting or energy clearing rituals, help release unhealthy attachments, promoting freedom, autonomy, and healthier energetic dynamics within relationships.

8. Enhancing Intimacy and Connection: Energy medicine offers practices to deepen intimacy and connection within relationships. Techniques such as couples' energy healing sessions, partner meditations, or tantric practices promote energetic attunement, heart-centered communication, and a sense of oneness. These practices foster a deeper sense of love, trust, and intimacy between partners.

9. Supporting Emotional Resilience: Emotional well-being is crucial for healthy relationships. Energy medicine techniques, including Emotional Freedom Techniques (EFT), chakra balancing, or energy grounding exercises, can support emotional resilience and regulation within relationships. By addressing emotional imbalances, individuals can cultivate emotional awareness, respond to challenges with greater clarity, and maintain healthier emotional boundaries.

10. Cultivating Positive Relationship Patterns: Energy medicine empowers individuals to consciously create positive relationship patterns. Through visualization, affirmation, and energy-clearing techniques, individuals can release negative relationship patterns and cultivate new energetic templates for healthy and fulfilling relationships. This promotes a positive energetic resonance and attracts relationships that are aligned with one's highest well-being.

11. Creating Sacred Space and Relationship Rituals: Creating sacred space and engaging in relationship rituals can deepen connection and strengthen the energetic bond between individuals

Energy medicine for couples

Relationships are a journey of growth, love, and connection, but they also require effort and care to thrive. Energy medicine offers a unique approach to supporting couples in deepening their bond, enhancing communication, and nurturing their relationship. By recognizing and working with the subtle energies that flow between partners, energy medicine practices can create a foundation for a fulfilling and harmonious partnership. Below we will explore the role of energy medicine in supporting couples, highlighting its benefits, considerations, and practical applications.

2. Energetic Awareness: Energy medicine emphasizes the importance of cultivating energetic awareness in relationships. Each individual carries their own unique energy, and when two people come together, their energies interact and intertwine. By developing awareness of our own energy and the energy of our partner, we can better understand the energetic dynamics within the relationship.

3. Enhancing Communication: Effective communication is vital for healthy relationships. Energy medicine practices can enhance communi-

cation by promoting active listening, empathy, and heart-centered connection. Techniques such as energy grounding exercises, mindful communication, or partner meditation can deepen understanding and strengthen the connection between couples.

4. Balancing Energetic Polarities: In any partnership, there are energetic polarities at play. Energy medicine recognizes the importance of balancing these polarities to create harmony within the relationship. Techniques such as chakra balancing, energy clearing, or polarity integration exercises can help partners align their energies and create a more balanced and harmonious energetic exchange.

5. Healing Relationship Wounds: Past wounds or unresolved emotional traumas can impact the dynamics of a relationship. Energy medicine provides tools to heal these wounds and create a safe and nurturing space for growth. Energy healing, guided visualization, or emotional release techniques can support couples in releasing old patterns and fostering healing within their relationship.

6. Cultivating Intimacy and Connection: Energy medicine practices can deepen intimacy and connection between partners. Techniques such as couples' energy healing sessions, shared meditation, or tantric practices promote energetic attunement, heart-centered connection, and a sense of oneness. These practices foster a deeper sense of love, trust, and intimacy within the relationship.

7. Clearing Energetic Blocks: Energetic blocks can hinder the flow of energy between partners and create disharmony. Energy medicine techniques, like Reiki, energy clearing rituals, or cord-cutting exercises, can help release these blocks and promote a more fluid and balanced energetic exchange. Clearing stagnant or negative energy allows for greater harmony and connection between partners.

8. Supporting Emotional Resilience: Emotional well-being is crucial for a healthy relationship. Energy medicine techniques, including Emotional Freedom Techniques (EFT), chakra balancing, or energy grounding exercises, can support emotional resilience within couples. By addressing emotional imbalances and promoting emotional awareness, partners can navigate challenges with greater clarity and maintain healthier emotional boundaries.

9. Creating Rituals and Sacred Space: Creating rituals and sacred space within the relationship fosters a sense of connection and deepens the energetic bond between partners. Energy medicine encourages couples to engage in practices such as shared meditation, energy-clearing rituals, or creating a sacred sanctuary within their home. These practices create a container for love, growth, and transformation within the relationship.

10. Nurturing Mutual Growth: Energy medicine recognizes that relationships are a catalyst for personal growth and transformation. Couples can support each other's growth by encouraging individual exploration of energy practices and sharing experiences. By supporting each other's journey, couples create an environment of mutual growth, understanding, and acceptance.

11. Rekindling Passion and Sensuality: Energy medicine techniques can reignite passion and sensuality within a relationship. Practices such as energy-boosting exercises, sensory awareness activities, or partner massage can enhance the energetic connection

Healing from toxic relationships and energy attachments

Toxic relationships can have a profound impact on our well-being, draining our energy, and hindering our personal growth. These relationships often leave energetic imprints and attachments that can continue to affect us long after the relationship has ended. Energy medicine provides valuable tools and practices to support the healing process, helping individuals release energetic attachments, restore balance, and reclaim their vitality. Below we will explore the role of energy medicine in healing from toxic relationships, highlighting its benefits, considerations, and practical applications.

2. Understanding Energetic Attachments: Energy medicine recognizes that toxic relationships can create energetic attachments between individuals. These attachments may manifest as energetic cords, imprints, or lingering emotional ties. Understanding the nature of these attachments is crucial for healing and moving forward.

3. Releasing Energetic Cords: Energetic cords are energetic connections that can form between individuals, particularly in toxic relationships. Energy medicine techniques, such as cord-cutting exercises, visualization, or energy clearing rituals, help release these cords and restore a sense of energetic autonomy. By consciously releasing the cords, individuals can break free from the energetic entanglement and regain their personal power.

4. Clearing Energetic Imprints: Toxic relationships leave energetic imprints that can impact our emotional well-being and energetic balance. Energy medicine practices, such as energy healing, aura cleansing, or guided visualization, facilitate the release of these imprints. By clearing the energetic residue of the toxic relationship, individuals can create space for healing and personal growth.

5. Restoring Energetic Boundaries: Toxic relationships often blur boundaries, leaving individuals energetically vulnerable. Energy medicine offers techniques to restore and strengthen energetic boundaries. Practices such as aura protection exercises, grounding techniques, or energy shielding can

support individuals in maintaining healthy boundaries, preventing further energy drain, and promoting self-protection.

6. Rebalancing the Energy Field: Toxic relationships can disrupt the balance of the energy field, leading to physical, emotional, and spiritual imbalances. Energy medicine approaches, including chakra balancing, energy clearing rituals, or energy healing, help rebalance the energy field, restoring harmony and vitality. By addressing the energetic imbalances, individuals can support their overall well-being and accelerate the healing process.

7. Emotional Release and Healing: Toxic relationships often leave emotional scars that require healing. Energy medicine provides techniques to support emotional release and healing, such as Emotional Freedom Techniques (EFT), breathwork, or somatic experiencing. These practices facilitate the release of trapped emotions, promote emotional healing, and restore emotional resilience.

8. Cultivating Self-Love and Self-Care: Healing from toxic relationships involves nurturing self-love and prioritizing self-care. Energy medicine encourages individuals to engage in practices that promote self-nurturing, such as self-massage, energy grounding exercises, or self-compassion meditations. By cultivating self-love and self-care, individuals strengthen their energetic foundation, restore their sense of worthiness, and create a solid platform for healing.

9. Supportive Therapies and Guidance: Healing from toxic relationships may require additional support from therapists, counselors, or energy healers experienced in working with trauma and energy dynamics. These professionals can provide guidance, support, and personalized energy medicine techniques tailored to the individual's specific needs.

10. Reconnecting with Authentic Self: Toxic relationships often lead to a disconnection from one's authentic self. Energy medicine practices, such

as meditation, mindfulness, or journaling, help individuals reconnect with their true essence. By aligning with their authentic self, individuals can rediscover their values, passions, and innate worth, facilitating the healing process.

11. Cultivating Positive Energies and Relationships: As individuals heal from toxic relationships, energy medicine

Chapter Seventeen

Self-Care and Energy Medicine

In our fast-paced and demanding world, self-care has become increasingly important for maintaining overall well-being and balance. Energy medicine offers a unique perspective on self-care, recognizing that our energetic state profoundly impacts our physical, emotional, and spiritual health. By incorporating energy medicine practices into our self-care routines, we can cultivate a deeper sense of well-being, rejuvenation, and harmony. Below we will explore the relationship between self-care and energy medicine, highlighting its benefits, considerations, and practical applications.

2. Understanding Energetic Self-Care: Energetic self-care involves nurturing and balancing our subtle energy systems, which include chakras, meridians, and the auric field. Energy medicine recognizes that disruptions or imbalances in these energy systems can lead to physical, emotional, and spiritual disharmony. Engaging in energetic self-care practices helps restore balance and promote overall well-being.

3. Daily Energy Hygiene: Just as we practice daily physical hygiene, it is equally essential to maintain daily energy hygiene. Energy medicine techniques, such as energy clearing rituals, self-massage, or aura cleansing exercises, can be incorporated into our daily self-care routines. These practices help remove energetic debris, refresh our energy field, and promote a sense of renewal and vitality.

4. Grounding and Centering: Grounding is an essential self-care practice that helps us stay connected to the Earth's energy and maintain stability amidst the demands of daily life. Energy medicine offers grounding exercises, visualization techniques, or nature walks to support grounding and centering. By grounding ourselves, we create a foundation of stability and balance, enhancing our overall well-being.

5. Energetic Protection: Energetic protection is a fundamental aspect of self-care, especially in environments where we may encounter negativity or energetic imbalances. Energy medicine practices, such as energy shielding, intention setting, or wearing protective crystals, help establish energetic boundaries and shield us from external influences that may drain our energy. By maintaining energetic protection, we can preserve our vitality and well-being.

6. Meditation and Mindfulness: Meditation and mindfulness practices are integral to energy medicine and self-care. These practices allow us to quiet the mind, cultivate inner peace, and connect with our deeper selves. Energy medicine offers various meditation techniques, breathwork exercises, or guided visualizations that promote relaxation, emotional balance, and spiritual growth.

7. Energy Healing and Rejuvenation: Energy healing modalities, such as Reiki, Quantum Touch, or Healing Touch, are powerful tools for self-care. These practices involve the gentle manipulation and balancing of the body's energy systems, promoting deep relaxation, stress reduction, and overall rejuvenation. By engaging in energy healing, we support our body's natural healing processes and enhance our well-being.

8. Emotional Release and Balancing: Emotional well-being is an essential aspect of self-care. Energy medicine techniques, including Emotional Freedom Techniques (EFT), energy psychology, or chakra balancing, facil-

itate the release of emotional blockages, promote emotional balance, and support mental clarity. By addressing and releasing suppressed emotions, we create space for healing, personal growth, and increased resilience.

9. Sacred Rituals and Self-Nurturing: Energy medicine encourages the incorporation of sacred rituals and self-nurturing practices into our self-care routines. These may include creating a sacred space for reflection, journaling, practicing gratitude, or engaging in self-massage with essential oils. These rituals promote self-love, self-compassion, and connection with our inner selves.

10. Intuitive Development: Cultivating our intuition is an important aspect of energy medicine and self-care. By developing our intuitive abilities, we can navigate life with greater clarity and make choices that align with our

Developing a daily energy medicine practice

In our quest for holistic well-being, incorporating energy medicine into our daily lives can be transformative. Energy medicine encompasses various practices that work with the subtle energies within and around us, promoting balance, vitality, and overall health. By developing a daily energy medicine practice, we can cultivate a deeper connection with our energetic selves and enhance our physical, emotional, and spiritual well-being. Below we will explore the benefits, considerations, and practical applications of developing a daily energy medicine practice.

2. Understanding Energy Medicine: Energy medicine recognizes that everything in the universe is composed of energy, including our bodies, thoughts, and emotions. By working with the subtle energies that flow within and around us, we can promote balance and well-being. Energy

medicine practices include modalities such as Reiki, acupuncture, qigong, chakra balancing, and many others.

3. Setting Intention: Developing a daily energy medicine practice begins with setting clear intentions. Determine the specific goals or areas of focus for your practice, such as reducing stress, promoting vitality, enhancing emotional well-being, or increasing spiritual connection. Setting intentions helps direct the energy and focus of your practice.

4. Grounding and Centering: Grounding and centering practices provide a solid foundation for energy work. Techniques such as walking barefoot in nature, standing or sitting with focused awareness on the connection to the Earth, or visualization exercises can help anchor your energy and bring you into the present moment. Grounding and centering promote stability, clarity, and balance.

5. Breathwork and Meditation: Incorporating breathwork and meditation into your daily energy medicine practice can have profound effects on your overall well-being. These practices calm the mind, reduce stress, and enhance energetic flow. Explore different meditation techniques such as mindfulness meditation, loving-kindness meditation, or guided visualization to find the methods that resonate with you.

6. Energetic Clearing: Energetic clearing practices help release stagnant or negative energy from your system, allowing for a more harmonious flow of energy. Techniques such as smudging with sage, using sound healing tools like singing bowls or tuning forks, or visualizing a cleansing white light can clear your energy field and promote a sense of renewal.

7. Chakra Balancing: Chakras are energy centers within our bodies that regulate the flow of energy. Balancing the chakras is essential for maintaining overall energetic harmony. Explore chakra balancing techniques, such as meditation focused on each chakra, working with corresponding

colors, or using crystals aligned with each chakra. Regular chakra balancing promotes vitality and supports emotional and physical well-being.

8. Self-Healing and Energy Touch: Self-healing practices allow you to become an active participant in your energy medicine practice. Reiki self-healing, acupressure, or tapping techniques like Emotional Freedom Techniques (EFT) can help restore energetic balance and alleviate physical and emotional discomfort. These practices empower you to take charge of your own healing journey.

9. Intuitive Development: Developing your intuition is an integral part of energy medicine practice. Trusting your intuition helps guide your energy work and enhances your connection with your energetic self. Engage in activities that foster intuitive development, such as journaling, meditation, or working with oracle cards. Developing your intuition expands your awareness and deepens your energetic practice.

10. Affirmations and Positive Intentions: Positive affirmations and intentions can shape the energy field and influence your overall well-being. Use affirmations that resonate with your goals and desires, and repeat them with conviction and positivity. Affirmations can help reprogram negative thought patterns and promote positive energy flow.

11. Reflective Practice: A daily energy medicine practice thrives on self-reflection and self-aware

Energy medicine for self-love and self-compassion

Self-love and self-compassion are vital components of our emotional well-being and overall happiness. They allow us to cultivate a deep sense of acceptance, kindness, and understanding toward ourselves. Energy medicine offers powerful tools and practices that can support the development of self-love and self-compassion, helping us foster inner harmony, heal emotional wounds, and nurture our well-being. Below we will explore the benefits, considerations, and practical applications of using energy medicine to enhance self-love and self-compassion.

2. Embracing the Energy of Love: Energy medicine recognizes that love is a powerful and transformative energy. By consciously connecting with the energy of love, we can cultivate self-love and self-compassion. Energy medicine practices, such as heart-centered meditations, affirmations, or energy healing techniques, help us tap into the loving energy within and around us.

3. Clearing Emotional Blocks: Emotional blocks and past traumas can hinder our ability to love and accept ourselves fully. Energy medicine provides tools to release these emotional blocks and promote emotional healing. Techniques such as Emotional Freedom Techniques (EFT), chakra balancing, or energy healing can support the release of negative emotions and foster a greater sense of self-compassion.

4. Chakra Balancing: Chakras are energy centers within our bodies that regulate the flow of energy. Balancing the chakras is essential for promoting self-love and self-compassion. Energy medicine offers practices to balance and harmonize the chakras, such as visualization, meditation, or energy healing. Balanced chakras facilitate the flow of loving energy and support emotional well-being.

5. Energetic Self-Care: Engaging in regular energetic self-care is a powerful act of self-love and self-compassion. Energy medicine practices, such as aura cleansing, energy clearing rituals, or self-massage with essential oils, help nurture our energetic well-being. By taking care of our energy, we show ourselves kindness and create a strong foundation for self-love.

6. Heart-Centered Practices: The heart is the center of love and compassion within us. Energy medicine emphasizes heart-centered practices that open our hearts and deepen our connection to ourselves. Techniques such as heart coherence meditation, sending love to ourselves through visualization, or practicing loving-kindness meditation foster self-love and self-compassion.

7. Forgiveness and Letting Go: Energy medicine recognizes the transformative power of forgiveness in cultivating self-love and self-compassion. Forgiving ourselves and others releases the energetic burden and promotes healing. Energy techniques like cord-cutting, visualization, or journaling can support the forgiveness process, allowing us to let go of past hurts and embrace self-compassion.

8. Affirmations and Positive Self-Talk: Affirmations and positive self-talk are effective tools for cultivating self-love and self-compassion. By consciously choosing positive thoughts and affirmations, we reprogram negative self-perceptions and build a supportive inner dialogue. Energy medicine encourages the use of affirmations, spoken or written, to promote self-love and acceptance.

9. Inner Child Healing: Our inner child carries the memories and emotions of our past experiences. Energy medicine offers techniques to heal and nurture our inner child, fostering self-love and self-compassion. Inner child meditations, energy healing, or creative visualization exercises can help address emotional wounds and reconnect with our innate sense of love and worthiness.

10. Gratitude Practice: Gratitude is a powerful practice that shifts our focus toward appreciation and love. Energy medicine encourages the cultivation of a daily gratitude practice to enhance self-love and self-compassion. By acknowledging the

Cultivating mindfulness and presence with energy medicine

In our fast-paced and often hectic lives, cultivating mindfulness and presence is essential for our well-being. Mindfulness allows us to be fully present in the moment, bringing our attention to the here and now. Energy medicine offers valuable tools and practices that can enhance our ability to cultivate mindfulness and presence, helping us deepen our connection with ourselves, others, and the world around us. Below we will explore the benefits, considerations, and practical applications of using energy medicine to cultivate mindfulness and presence.

2. Understanding Mindfulness and Presence: Mindfulness involves intentionally bringing our attention to the present moment without judgment. It involves observing our thoughts, emotions, and sensations as they arise, allowing us to fully experience and engage with our present reality. Energy medicine recognizes that mindfulness and presence are not only mental states but also energetic states that can be cultivated and enhanced.

3. Conscious Breathing: Breath is a powerful tool for cultivating mindfulness and presence. Energy medicine emphasizes the importance of conscious breathing, as it helps us anchor our attention to the present moment and connect with our life force energy. Breathing techniques, such as deep belly breathing or alternate nostril breathing, can support our ability to be fully present.

4. Grounding and Centering: Grounding and centering practices are foundational for cultivating mindfulness and presence. By grounding ourselves, we establish a connection with the Earth's energy, which helps us stay rooted in the present moment. Energy medicine offers grounding

exercises, visualization techniques, or nature walks to support grounding and centering.

5. Body Awareness: Energy medicine recognizes that the body is a powerful vehicle for experiencing the present moment. Cultivating body awareness through practices such as body scanning, yoga, or tai chi allows us to connect with our physical sensations and deepen our presence. By tuning into the body's energy, we can become more attuned to the present moment.

6. Energetic Sensitivity: Energy medicine encourages the development of energetic sensitivity, which involves becoming aware of the subtle energy that flows within and around us. By honing our energetic sensitivity, we can sense the subtle shifts in energy and become more present in our interactions and experiences. Energetic practices, such as Reiki, qigong, or aura scanning, can enhance our ability to perceive and work with energy.

7. Mindful Movement: Engaging in mindful movement practices, such as walking meditation, yoga, or qigong, can deepen our connection with the present moment. Energy medicine acknowledges the transformative power of mindful movement in balancing our energy, calming the mind, and cultivating presence. By bringing awareness to each movement and sensation, we enhance our mindfulness practice.

8. Energetic Boundaries: Maintaining clear energetic boundaries is crucial for cultivating mindfulness and presence. Energy medicine offers techniques for establishing and maintaining healthy boundaries, such as energy shielding, visualization, or intention setting. By setting energetic boundaries, we create a sense of safety and protection, allowing us to fully be present in the moment.

9. Energy Healing and Presence: Energy healing modalities, such as Reiki or Healing Touch, promote deep relaxation and energetic balance. When

receiving energy healing, we are encouraged to be fully present and receptive, allowing the healing energy to flow through us. This practice enhances our capacity for presence and deepens our connection with the energetic aspect of ourselves.

10. Mindful Eating: Energy medicine emphasizes the importance of mindful eating, which involves bringing full awareness to the experience of eating. By engaging all our senses and savoring each bite, we cultivate presence and appreciation for the nourishment we receive. Mindful eating supports our overall well-being and fosters a deeper connection with our body and its energy.

11. Energy Meditation: Energy meditation practices go beyond

Chapter Eighteen

Energy Medicine and the Environment

Energy medicine offers more than just personal healing and well-being; it also holds the potential to create positive change in the world around us. As we explore the interconnectedness of all beings and the environment, we begin to understand the profound impact our energy has on the Earth. By aligning our energy practices with environmental consciousness, we can promote healing, sustainability, and harmony. Below we will explore the relationship between energy medicine and the environment, highlighting the ways in which our energetic practices can contribute to a healthier planet.

2. The Interconnectedness of All Beings: Energy medicine recognizes that all beings are interconnected and share an energetic bond with the Earth. Our well-being is intricately linked to the health and vitality of the environment. By understanding this interconnectedness, we can foster a deeper sense of responsibility for the Earth's well-being.

3. Healing the Earth's Energy: Just as energy medicine focuses on balancing and harmonizing our personal energy, it can also be applied to healing the energy of the Earth. Practices such as Earth healing ceremonies, sending healing energy to natural environments, or working with Earth element energies help restore balance and vitality to the Earth's energetic systems.

4. Energy Awareness and Conservation: Energy medicine encourages us to cultivate awareness of our personal energy consumption and make

conscious choices that promote sustainability. By conserving energy, reducing waste, and choosing renewable energy sources, we contribute to the preservation of the Earth's resources and lessen our impact on the environment.

5. Environmental Stewardship: Energy medicine practitioners can become environmental stewards, advocating for sustainable practices and raising awareness about the impact of human activities on the environment. By sharing knowledge and promoting eco-friendly initiatives, we inspire others to take action and become conscious custodians of the Earth.

6. Energetic Space Clearing: Energy medicine practices can be applied to clear and harmonize the energy of physical spaces, including homes, workplaces, and natural environments. By engaging in energetic space clearing techniques, such as smudging, sound healing, or intention setting, we create energetically supportive environments that promote healing and balance.

7. Connecting with Nature: Energy medicine encourages us to connect with nature as a source of healing and inspiration. Spending time in natural settings, such as forests, mountains, or bodies of water, allows us to attune to the Earth's energy and experience the profound interconnectedness of all living beings. This connection deepens our appreciation for the environment and fuels our desire to protect it.

8. Plant and Animal Energies: Energy medicine acknowledges the wisdom and healing properties of plants and animals. By working with plant essences, herbal remedies, or animal spirit guides, we tap into the healing energy of nature and deepen our connection with the natural world. Respectful and sustainable practices are essential when using plant and animal energies to ensure their preservation.

9. Conscious Consumption: Energy medicine invites us to approach consumption with mindfulness and conscious awareness. By making informed choices about the products we use and their impact on the environment, we reduce our carbon footprint and support sustainable industries. This includes opting for organic and eco-friendly products, reducing single-use items, and supporting local and ethical businesses.

10. Collective Energy Healing: Energy medicine practitioners can come together to participate in collective energy healing practices focused on the environment. These may include group meditations, prayers, or ceremonies dedicated to planetary healing. By amplifying our collective intention and energy, we contribute to the restoration and well-being of the Earth.

11. Teaching Energy Medicine and Environmental Awareness: As practitioners of energy medicine, we have the opportunity to teach others about the importance of environmental awareness and how energy practices can positively impact the planet. By sharing our knowledge and skills, we empower individuals to become agents of change and engage in

The impact of environmental factors on the energy body

The environment in which we live plays a significant role in shaping our physical, emotional, and energetic well-being. Our energy bodies, as recognized in energy medicine, are influenced by various environmental factors, ranging from natural elements to human-made surroundings. Understanding the interplay between these factors and the energy body can deepen our awareness and guide us in maintaining balance and vitality. Below we will explore the impact of environmental factors on the energy body and their relevance in the context of energy medicine.

2. Natural Elements: Nature has a profound influence on our energy bodies. The air we breathe, the sunlight that nourishes us, the earth beneath our feet, and the water we drink all contribute to our energetic balance. Fresh air, abundant sunlight, grounding with the Earth, and exposure to natural bodies of water positively impact our energy bodies and promote overall well-being.

3. Geographical Location: The geographical location in which we reside can affect our energy bodies in various ways. Different regions have unique energy signatures, such as ley lines, vortexes, or geopathic stress. Energy medicine practitioners often consider the energetic qualities of specific locations and their impact on individuals' energy bodies. Harmonizing with the energy of a particular place can enhance our energetic well-being.

4. Electromagnetic Fields (EMFs): In today's modern world, we are exposed to electromagnetic fields emitted by electronic devices, power lines, and wireless technology. Prolonged exposure to high levels of EMFs can disrupt the energy flow within our bodies, leading to imbalances and potential health concerns. Energy medicine techniques, such as grounding exercises, shielding, and minimizing exposure to EMFs, can help mitigate their impact on the energy body.

5. Architecture and Building Materials: The structures we inhabit can influence our energy bodies. The design, layout, and materials used in buildings can impact the flow of energy within a space. Energy medicine practitioners may assess the energetic qualities of a building and offer recommendations for creating a harmonious environment that supports the energy body. Incorporating natural materials, optimizing natural light, and creating energetically balanced spaces can positively affect our well-being.

6. Environmental Toxins: Exposure to environmental toxins, such as air pollution, chemicals, and heavy metals, can disrupt the energy flow in our bodies. These toxins can accumulate in our energy centers, compromising their function and overall energy balance. Energy medicine practices, such as detoxification techniques, energy clearing, and supporting the body's natural detox pathways, help mitigate the impact of environmental toxins on the energy body.

7. Colors and Vibrations: Colors have distinct energetic vibrations that can affect our energy bodies. Certain colors may promote balance and harmony, while others can stimulate or calm specific energy centers. Energy medicine utilizes color therapy, where individuals are exposed to specific colors to promote energetic balance and well-being. This can involve wearing certain colors, visualizing colors during meditation, or incorporating colored objects in our environment.

8. Sound and Vibrations: Sound has a profound effect on our energy bodies. Harmonious sounds, such as calming music, nature sounds, or chanting, can positively influence our energetic state, promoting relaxation and balance. Energy medicine practitioners may utilize sound healing techniques, such as singing bowls, tuning forks, or vocal toning, to restore energetic harmony within the body.

9. Nature Connection: Establishing a deep connection with nature has a transformative impact on our energy bodies. Spending time in natural surroundings, engaging in activities like forest bathing, hiking, or gardening, allows us to align with the Earth's natural rhythms and recharge our energy. The energy medicine perspective acknowledges the vital role nature plays in supporting our energetic well-being.

10. Climate and Seasonal Changes: Climate and seasonal variations can affect our

Energy medicine for space clearing and creating a healing environment

The spaces we inhabit hold energetic imprints that can impact our well-being and overall harmony. Energy medicine offers valuable techniques for space clearing and creating healing environments, allowing us to optimize the energetic flow and promote a sense of balance, peace, and vitality. Below we will explore the concept of space clearing in relation to energy medicine and delve into practical applications for creating healing spaces.

2. Understanding Energetic Imprints: Energy medicine recognizes that spaces can hold energetic imprints from past events, emotions, or interactions. These imprints can affect the energetic flow within a space and impact the well-being of its occupants. By acknowledging and addressing these imprints, we can create a fresh energetic foundation that supports healing and harmony.

3. Intention Setting: Intention is a powerful tool in energy medicine and space clearing. By setting a clear and positive intention for the space, we can direct the energy toward healing and transformation. Intention setting can be done through meditation, visualization, or affirmation, allowing us to infuse the space with our desired energetic qualities.

4. Energy Clearing Techniques: Energy medicine offers various techniques for clearing stagnant or negative energy from a space. Smudging with sage or other herbs, using sound healing tools like bells or singing bowls, and performing energy clearing rituals can help remove energetic blockages and restore the flow of positive energy.

5. Energetic Grids and Layout: Energy medicine recognizes the importance of the energetic grid and layout of a space. The placement of furniture, objects, and decor can either support or hinder the flow of energy.

By harmonizing the arrangement of elements within a space, we create an energetic grid that promotes balance, clarity, and well-being.

6. Feng Shui: Feng Shui, an ancient Chinese practice, is closely related to energy medicine and space clearing. It involves harmonizing the energy flow within a space by considering factors such as furniture placement, color schemes, and the five elements (wood, fire, earth, metal, and water). Feng Shui principles help create a balanced and harmonious environment that supports health and well-being.

7. Crystals and Stones: Crystals and stones are known for their energetic properties and can be used in space clearing to enhance positive energy flow. Placing crystals strategically within a space can help transmute negative energy and infuse the area with positive vibrations. Each crystal has its unique qualities, and choosing crystals that align with the desired energy can amplify the healing potential of a space.

8. Natural Elements: Incorporating natural elements in a space contributes to its healing energy. Plants, flowers, natural light, and flowing water introduce organic and vibrant energy into the environment. Energy medicine encourages the inclusion of natural elements as they promote a connection to the Earth and infuse the space with life force energy.

9. Color Therapy: Colors have specific energetic frequencies that can influence the mood and energy of a space. Energy medicine considers color therapy in space clearing by using specific colors to create a desired energetic atmosphere. Warm colors like red or orange can invigorate and stimulate, while cool colors like blue or green can create a calming and soothing ambiance.

10. Sacred Space Creation: Creating a sacred space within a larger environment is a powerful way to cultivate a healing environment. A sacred space can be a dedicated corner, altar, or room where one can engage in

spiritual practices, meditation, or reflection. By intentionally consecrating and maintaining a sacred space, we invite positive energies and create a sanctuary for rejuvenation and introspection.

11. Regular Maintenance: Regularly maintaining the energetic cleanliness of a space is essential for ongoing well-being. Energy medicine emphasizes the importance of regular space clearing practices to ensure a balanced and harmonious environment

Techniques for protecting your energy in challenging environments

In today's fast-paced and demanding world, we often find ourselves in challenging environments that can drain our energy and impact our overall well-being. However, energy medicine offers valuable techniques for protecting our energy and maintaining balance even in the most difficult situations. By cultivating awareness and implementing effective practices, we can navigate challenging environments with resilience and protect our energetic vitality. Below we will explore techniques for protecting your energy in challenging environments, drawing from the principles of energy medicine.

2. Grounding and Centering: Grounding is a foundational practice in energy medicine that helps us establish a connection with the Earth's energy, providing stability and balance. When faced with challenging environments, grounding and centering techniques, such as visualizations, deep breathing, or engaging with nature, can help anchor our energy, keeping us rooted and resilient.

3. Energetic Boundaries: Energetic boundaries act as a protective shield, preserving our energy and preventing external influences from overwhelming us. Energy medicine emphasizes the importance of setting clear

boundaries, both physically and energetically. Techniques such as visualization, intention setting, and working with protective symbols or crystals can help establish and maintain healthy boundaries in challenging environments.

4. Shielding: Shielding is a practice that involves creating an energetic barrier around oneself to shield against negative or draining energies. This technique can be particularly useful in challenging environments where there is a high concentration of stress or negativity. Visualizations of a protective shield, invoking the energy of light, or working with specific shielding techniques from energy medicine modalities can provide effective protection.

5. Conscious Energy Awareness: Developing conscious energy awareness allows us to recognize when our energy is being affected in challenging environments. Energy medicine emphasizes the importance of self-observation and tuning into our energy. By paying attention to physical sensations, emotions, and subtle energetic shifts, we can identify when our energy is being depleted or compromised, enabling us to take appropriate measures to protect and restore our vitality.

6. Energy Clearing: Regular energy clearing practices are vital for releasing any negative or stagnant energy that may accumulate in challenging environments. Techniques such as smudging, bathing or showering with intention, or visualization exercises can help cleanse and restore our energy, ensuring we are not carrying the energetic residue of challenging environments within us.

7. Mindful Awareness of Surroundings: Being mindful of our surroundings is crucial in challenging environments. Energy medicine encourages us to observe the energetic qualities of the spaces we occupy, including the people, objects, and overall atmosphere. By cultivating awareness, we

can make conscious choices about the environments we expose ourselves to and take necessary precautions to protect our energy when faced with challenging circumstances.

8. Self-Care Practices: Self-care is essential for maintaining our energetic well-being, especially in challenging environments. Engaging in activities that nourish and rejuvenate us, such as meditation, journaling, exercise, or spending time in nature, replenishes our energy reserves and enhances our resilience. Energy medicine encourages the integration of self-care practices as an integral part of protecting and nurturing our energy.

9. Emotional Regulation: Challenging environments often evoke strong emotions that can impact our energy. Energy medicine emphasizes the importance of emotional regulation techniques, such as breathwork, meditation, or journaling, to process and release challenging emotions. By addressing emotional reactions effectively, we can prevent our energy from being drained or depleted in these environments.

10. Positive Affirmations and Mantras: Positive affirmations and mantras are powerful tools in energy medicine for cultivating a positive mindset and protecting our energy. By affirming our worthiness, setting intentions for positive experiences, or reciting empowering mantras, we shift our energetic vibration and create a protective energetic shield that rep

Chapter Nineteen

Professional Development in Energy Medicine

Energy medicine is a rapidly evolving field that offers a wealth of opportunities for professional development and growth. As more individuals recognize the power of energy-based healing modalities, the demand for skilled practitioners continues to grow. Whether you are just starting your journey in energy medicine or seeking to advance your existing practice, investing in professional development is essential for staying current, expanding your skill set, and providing the best possible care to your clients. Below we will explore the significance of professional development in energy medicine and discuss various avenues for nurturing growth and excellence in the field.

2. Continual Learning: Energy medicine is a dynamic and multidisciplinary field, and there is always something new to learn. Engaging in continual learning through workshops, seminars, courses, and conferences helps you stay updated on the latest research, techniques, and advancements in energy medicine. By expanding your knowledge base, you can offer a broader range of treatments and insights to your clients.

3. Specialization and Advanced Training: As energy medicine encompasses various modalities and approaches, specializing in a specific area of interest can enhance your expertise and credibility. Pursuing advanced training in a particular modality, such as Reiki, acupuncture, or sound healing, allows you to develop a deeper understanding and proficiency in

that specific practice. Specialization also enables you to better serve clients with specific needs or interests.

4. Mentorship and Supervision: Seeking mentorship or supervision from experienced practitioners in energy medicine can provide invaluable guidance and support. Mentors can share their wisdom, offer feedback on your practice, and help you navigate challenges that arise in your professional journey. Their insights can help you refine your skills, deepen your understanding, and gain confidence as a practitioner.

5. Research and Evidence-Based Practice: Energy medicine is increasingly gaining recognition in the scientific and medical communities. Engaging in research and integrating evidence-based practices in your work helps solidify the credibility of energy medicine as a legitimate healing modality. By staying informed about current research, conducting your own studies, or collaborating with researchers, you contribute to the growth and acceptance of energy medicine as a valid approach to healthcare.

6. Ethical and Professional Standards: Upholding ethical and professional standards is paramount in the field of energy medicine. Adhering to a code of ethics ensures that you provide safe and responsible care to your clients while maintaining confidentiality and respecting their autonomy. Continuing education on ethical guidelines and professional standards helps you navigate ethical dilemmas and make informed decisions in your practice.

7. Collaborative Networking: Building a network of like-minded professionals in energy medicine offers numerous benefits. Engaging in collaborative networking provides opportunities for knowledge exchange, skill sharing, and professional support. Collaborative projects, research studies, or joint workshops with colleagues can enhance your professional development and broaden your impact in the field.

8. Continuing Professional Education (CPE) Requirements: Many professional organizations and regulatory bodies in energy medicine have CPE requirements to maintain certification or licensure. These requirements ensure that practitioners remain current in their knowledge and skills. Fulfilling CPE requirements through approved courses, workshops, or self-study programs ensures ongoing growth and competence in your practice.

9. Supervised Practice and Case Studies: Engaging in supervised practice and conducting case studies allows you to refine your skills and gain practical experience under the guidance of experienced professionals. Supervised practice provides opportunities to receive feedback, fine-tune your techniques, and ensure the highest level of care for your clients. Documenting and analyzing case studies helps expand your understanding of the efficacy of energy medicine techniques and allows you to contribute to the body of knowledge in the field.

10. Professional Associations and Memberships: Joining professional associations or organizations in the field of energy medicine provides a supportive community and access to valuable resources.

Finding the right energy medicine modality for you

Energy medicine encompasses a wide range of modalities and practices that aim to restore balance and promote well-being on an energetic level. With numerous options available, finding the right energy medicine modality for you can be an exciting and transformative journey. Each modality offers unique approaches, techniques, and philosophies, allowing individuals to explore and connect with the modality that resonates most with their needs and interests. Below we will delve into the process of finding the right energy medicine modality for you, highlighting key considerations and pathways to healing and growth.

2. Self-Reflection and Intention: Begin your exploration by reflecting on your personal needs, goals, and intentions for seeking energy medicine. Consider the specific areas of your life or well-being that you wish to address, such as physical health, emotional well-being, spiritual growth, or stress reduction. Clarifying your intentions will help guide your search for the right modality that aligns with your goals.

3. Research and Education: Engage in thorough research to familiarize yourself with different energy medicine modalities. Explore reputable resources, books, websites, and scientific literature to gain knowledge about the various approaches, techniques, and philosophies. Educate yourself on the principles, beliefs, and evidence supporting each modality to make informed decisions.

4. Seek Recommendations: Seek recommendations from trusted sources, such as healthcare professionals, friends, family, or colleagues who have personal experience with energy medicine. Their insights and recommendations can provide valuable guidance and help you narrow down your choices.

5. Consult with Practitioners: Schedule consultations or introductory sessions with practitioners of different energy medicine modalities. These sessions allow you to experience firsthand the techniques and approaches used in each modality. Discuss your specific concerns, goals, and expectations with the practitioners, and observe how their approach resonates with you. This firsthand experience will aid in determining whether a particular modality feels right for you.

6. Attend Workshops and Classes: Attend workshops, introductory classes, or community events that offer exposure to multiple energy medicine modalities. These immersive experiences provide a broader understanding of the different approaches and allow you to explore various techniques.

By participating in hands-on activities, you can gauge your comfort level and personal resonance with each modality.

7. Trust Your Intuition: Pay attention to your intuitive guidance when exploring energy medicine modalities. Your inner wisdom can often provide valuable insights and lead you toward the modality that feels most aligned with your needs. Trusting your intuition can help you navigate through the abundance of choices and find the modality that resonates deeply within you.

8. Personal Compatibility: Consider your personal preferences and comfort level when selecting an energy medicine modality. Some modalities may involve physical touch, while others may focus on energetic techniques without physical contact. Reflect on your comfort level with different approaches and determine what feels most appropriate for you.

9. Compatibility with Beliefs and Values: Consider the compatibility of the modality's philosophy and principles with your own beliefs and values. Energy medicine modalities may draw from diverse traditions, cultural practices, or spiritual frameworks. Assess whether the underlying principles of a particular modality align with your worldview and resonate with your personal beliefs.

10. Training and Accessibility: Evaluate the training requirements and accessibility of the modality you are interested in pursuing. Some modalities may require extensive training or certification, while others may offer more accessible entry points. Consider the time commitment, financial investment, and practicality of training in a specific modality, ensuring it aligns with your resources and lifestyle.

11. Personal Connection and Support: Pay attention to the personal connection and support you feel within the energy medicine modality.

Consider the availability of mentors, community support, or online resources that can

Training and certification options

Training and certification are essential aspects of developing expertise and credibility in the field of energy medicine. They provide individuals with the necessary knowledge, skills, and recognition to practice energy medicine effectively and ethically. As the demand for qualified practitioners continues to grow, a variety of training and certification options are available to support individuals in their journey towards becoming skilled energy medicine practitioners. Below we will explore the importance of training and certification in energy medicine, and discuss the various options and considerations for pursuing education and professional growth.

2. Establishing a Foundation: Training programs in energy medicine often begin by establishing a solid foundation in the principles and concepts underlying the modality. These foundational courses provide an understanding of energy systems, the interconnectedness of mind, body, and spirit, and the principles of energy healing. They equip students with a comprehensive understanding of the theoretical framework that guides energy medicine practices.

3. Hands-On Practical Experience: Alongside theoretical knowledge, practical experience is a crucial component of energy medicine training. Hands-on practice allows students to apply the learned concepts and techniques, honing their skills and gaining confidence. Practical experience can include supervised practice, case studies, and clinical placements, enabling students to integrate theory into real-life scenarios.

4. Specialized Modalities and Techniques: Energy medicine encompasses a wide range of modalities and techniques, each with its own unique

approach and focus. Training programs often offer specialized courses that delve deeper into specific modalities such as Reiki, acupuncture, or qigong, allowing individuals to develop expertise in their chosen area of interest. These specialized courses provide in-depth knowledge and practical skills required to practice specific modalities effectively.

5. Accredited Programs and Institutions: When selecting a training program in energy medicine, it is important to consider accreditation and recognition by relevant professional bodies or organizations. Accredited programs ensure that the curriculum meets specific standards of quality and adhere to ethical guidelines. Accreditation provides assurance that the training program is reputable and that the certification obtained is recognized within the field.

6. Certification and Licensing: Certification and licensing serve as formal recognition of competency and expertise in energy medicine. They provide credibility and assure clients that practitioners have met specific standards of training and practice. Certification requirements may vary depending on the modality and the governing body. Some modalities may have their own certification boards, while others may require certification through professional associations.

7. Continuing Education and Advanced Training: Energy medicine is a constantly evolving field, with new research, techniques, and practices emerging regularly. Pursuing continuing education and advanced training ensures that practitioners stay current and expand their knowledge and skills. Continuing education may involve attending workshops, conferences, or advanced training courses to deepen understanding and refine techniques.

8. Online and Distance Learning: The advent of technology has opened up opportunities for online and distance learning in energy medicine.

Online courses offer flexibility and convenience, allowing individuals to access training from anywhere in the world. These courses often include video lectures, interactive modules, and online forums for discussion and support. However, it is important to ensure that online programs are reputable and provide adequate practical training components.

9. Mentorship and Apprenticeship: Mentorship and apprenticeship programs provide valuable guidance and support as individuals progress in their energy medicine journey. Working closely with experienced practitioners allows students to gain insights, receive feedback, and develop their skills under the mentor's guidance. Mentorship programs often combine hands-on training, supervision, and personalized guidance.

10. Continuing Professional Development (CPD): Energy medicine practitioners are encouraged to engage in continuous professional development (CPD) to enhance their knowledge and skills. CPD can include attending conferences, participating in workshops, conducting research, or presenting at professional events. CPD ensures practitioners stay updated on advancements in the field and continue to provide high

Building a successful energy medicine practice

Building a successful energy medicine practice requires more than just technical expertise in healing modalities. It involves a combination of knowledge, skills, passion, and a deep understanding of the principles that underpin energy medicine. As an energy medicine practitioner, establishing a thriving practice allows you to make a meaningful impact on the well-being of your clients and the community. Below we will explore key considerations and strategies for building a successful energy medicine practice.

2. Develop Expertise and Specialization: To build a successful energy medicine practice, it is important to develop expertise and specialization in specific modalities or areas of interest. This specialization allows you to differentiate yourself and become known for your unique skills and offerings. Invest in advanced training, mentorship, and continuing education to deepen your knowledge and refine your techniques in your chosen specialization.

3. Establish a Solid Foundation: Building a successful energy medicine practice begins with establishing a solid foundation. Ensure you have a thorough understanding of the principles, ethics, and theoretical frameworks that guide energy medicine. Continually deepen your understanding through research, reading, and staying informed about the latest developments in the field. A strong foundation will provide the necessary confidence and credibility to attract and retain clients.

4. Create a Healing Space: The physical environment in which you practice energy medicine plays a vital role in client experience. Create a welcoming, calming, and energetically balanced space that fosters relaxation, healing, and trust. Pay attention to factors such as lighting, color schemes, comfortable furnishings, and the overall ambiance. Incorporate elements of nature, such as plants or natural materials, to enhance the healing environment.

5. Cultivate Effective Communication Skills: Effective communication is crucial in building a successful energy medicine practice. Develop excellent listening skills to understand clients' needs, concerns, and goals. Clearly articulate the benefits of energy medicine and explain complex concepts in simple, relatable terms. Establish open and honest communication, ensuring clients feel heard, understood, and supported throughout their healing journey.

6. Nurture Trust and Rapport: Building trust and rapport with clients is essential for a thriving practice. Create a safe, non-judgmental, and compassionate space where clients feel comfortable sharing their concerns and experiences. Maintain client confidentiality and establish clear professional boundaries. Cultivate a genuine sense of empathy, compassion, and respect for each client's unique journey.

7. Embrace Holistic Approaches: Energy medicine recognizes the interconnectedness of mind, body, and spirit. Embrace holistic approaches by considering the physical, emotional, mental, and spiritual aspects of your clients' well-being. Incorporate techniques that address the whole person, rather than focusing solely on symptomatic relief. Educate clients about the importance of self-care, lifestyle choices, and holistic practices that support their overall well-being.

8. Establish a Client-Centered Approach: Tailor your energy medicine practice to meet the specific needs and goals of your clients. Conduct thorough assessments to gain a comprehensive understanding of their individual circumstances. Develop customized treatment plans that integrate various energy medicine techniques and modalities to address their unique concerns. Regularly evaluate and adjust treatment plans based on clients' progress and feedback.

9. Emphasize Continuing Education and Growth: The field of energy medicine is constantly evolving. Emphasize continuing education and personal growth to stay current and enhance your practice. Attend workshops, conferences, and seminars to expand your knowledge, learn new techniques, and engage with the energy medicine community. Seek mentorship or supervision to receive guidance, support, and feedback on your practice.

10. Develop a Professional Network: Building a successful energy medicine practice involves developing a strong professional network. Collaborate with other healthcare professionals, complementary therapists, and practitioners in related fields. Establish mutually beneficial referral networks and attend networking events.

* 9 7 8 1 7 7 6 8 4 9 0 4 8 *

SD - #0043 - 140926 - C0 - 229/152/11 - PB - 9781776849048 - Matt Lamination